CORONOIA

What the W.H.O. failed to tell us and the UK Cabinet refused to hear

Dr Harley Farmer
PhD BVSc (Hons) BVBiol (Path) MRCVS

Foreword by Dr Kim A. Jobst
DM FRCP MFHom

To Dr Anne-Marie Farmer, my wife, who has guided me through challenging waters during our 43 wonderful years of married life.

Published in 2020 by NewGenne Ltd whose registered office is at: 4 Hereward Way Business Park, Harling Road, Roudham, Norfolk, NR16 2SR, UK.

© Dr Harley Farmer

For information about how to apply for permission to reuse the copyright material in this book and for customer services please see our website: www.newgenne.com. All unauthorised use of the copyright material in this book is strictly prohibited.

The right of the author to be identified as the author of this work has been asserted in accordance with the Copyright, Designs and Patents Act 1988.

Library of Congress Cataloging-in-Publication data

Farmer, Harley
Coronoia: What the WHO failed to tell us and the UK Cabinet refused to hear
ISBN 978-0-9569707-9-4

A catalogue record of this book is available from the British Library.

All rights reserved. No part of this publication may be produced, stored in a retrieval system, or transmitted, in any form or by any means, electronic, mechanical, photocopying, recording or otherwise, except as permitted by the UK Copyright, Designs and Patents Act 1988, without prior permission of the publisher.

Some material included with standard print versions of this book may not be included in e-books.

Disclaimer of Warranty / Limit of Liability: While the author and publisher have used their best efforts in preparing this book, they make no representations or warranties with respect to the accuracy or completeness of the contents of this book and specifically disclaim any implied warranties of merchantability or fitness for a particular purpose. It is sold or given on the understanding that the publisher and author are not engaged in rendering professional services and neither the publisher nor the author shall be liable for damages arising therefrom. If professional advice or other expert assistance is required, the services of a competent professional should be sought.

None of the information in this book is given as a diagnosis or recommendation for treatment and no implication of diagnosis or treatment recommendation should be made or implied.

The thesis on which this book is predicated is presented as a suggestion intended to be debated so the thesis can be either considered correct or disproved. The thesis is conjecture on the author's part and is not intended to be seen as fact, nor is it to be quoted or replicated as fact.

The information contained in this book is derived from reputable, authentic and highly regarded sources. Where that information is quoting published scientific and medical articles the full references from which the information is derived are provided in the bibliography at the end of this book.

Links to websites are liable to change if the owner of the website exercises their right to alter their website. If a link ceases to operate, the reader is asked to find the current link to the information if the latter is still being made available by the owner of the website. If websites referred to are subsequently removed from access the reader is asked to ignore references made in this text to such websites.

Trademark Notice: Application has been made to register Coronoia and NewGenne as trademarks with the intention of extending the trademarks to international jurisdictions. Trademarks or corporate names in the text may be trademarks or registered trademarks, and are used only for identification and explanation without intent to infringe.

This work was produced in collaboration with Write Business Results Limited. For more information on Write Business Results' business book, blog and podcast services, please visit www.writebusinessresults.com or email your query to info@writebusinessresults.com.

FOREWORD

Dr Kim A. Jobst DM FRCP MFHom

"We defy augury.
There's a special providence in the fall of a sparrow.
If it be now, 'tis not to come.
If it be not to come, it will be now.
If it be not now, yet it will come – the readiness is all."
Hamlet, Act 5, Scene 2

This book contains information that if understood, verified and acted upon will not only prevent the loss of many millions of lives but radically impact the economic, political and environmental future of our planet. This is no hyperbole as you will discover in what follows.

The reason for invoking Hamlet's timeless words at the outset contextualises the significance of this book, its content and its potential global impact. The words, "if it be not now, yet it will come – the readiness is all", make it clear that this book *will* have its impact ("yet it will come") even if not immediately now ("If it be not now"). The critical element is two-fold in that the readiness is expressed both in you and me being alert to every possible opportunity to influence and educate, as well as having, and acting with, the courage and foresight to stand out, share the truth as we see it, and advocate, in our own lives, changes that will affect buying and selling, and all the activities of life locally, nationally and internationally. If this work is proven correct the whole accelerated vaccination agenda might even be delayed for full and proper safety testing, for example. The ramifications are truly awe-inspiring and all follow from executing one very simple procedural change to how we execute and understand sanitisation.

Of all the hundreds of thousands of words I have read since the beginning of this SARS-CoV-2 (Covid-19) pandemic, those in this book by Dr Harley Farmer PhD MRCVS are amongst the most poignant and important of all. And they are deceptively profound in their simplicity and accessibility. As a physician-scientist dedicated to exploring and understanding what might enable people to heal, i.e. become whole, in body, mind and spirit, what Dr Harley Farmer has put together here, on the background of 20 years' work engaging with and overcoming viruses such as Noro, MERS and SARS-1, which if left unchecked can cause mayhem with disease, is of the order of Louis Pasteur and Joseph Lister. Pasteur proposed germ theory, and Lister, acting on what he learned from Pasteur, suggested that applying chemical agents as antiseptics in and around the surgeon's operating field, as well as on floors and surfaces, including hands and instruments, would save lives. In so doing he birthed the whole discipline of antisepsis and the industry that has ensued, which is currently at the centre of the thesis of this book. Today, germ theory has been proven to be causally involved in infection beyond all reasonable doubt. What gives rise to infection in one person over another who doesn't "catch" it, when two human beings, side by side, might be exposed to the same germs, remains a subject of profound debate and enquiry.

Whatever the case, germs/microbes that were at the time invisible to Pasteur and Lister were postulated to be the cause of infection, morbidity and mortality, as well as the active agents in the fermentation of wine and beer i.e. alcohol. Taking up Pasteur's work, Lister went on to work with antisepsis, dramatically reducing the death toll from surgery in the late 1800s, and transforming clinical practice. Lister, for all his genius, dedication, equanimity and seriousness about saving and maintaining life, was ridiculed, made the butt of disparaging jokes and referred to as "a pretentious charlatan" whose ideas were both foolish and dangerous. With what we know today about infection, that seems not just cruel but absurd. Yet at the time, for the what is invisible to be the cause of infection, festering wounds and death, so challenged the mind-set of the majority and flew in the face of accepted wisdom and theory, not least because it demanded of surgeons and practitioners a change in practice and a new way of clearing and cleaning treatment and operating fields. Take note – something that at the time was unseen (microbes/germs) was being postulated to be the cause of infection and death. The same is true in what is suggested in this book, as you will see; only in this story the unseen is a vapour arising from a ubiquitously used liquid sanitising agent – alcohol.

In my opinion, *Coronoia: What the WHO failed to tell us and the UK Cabinet refused to hear* is of an equivalent order to the work of those giants on whose shoulders we have learned to stand. They were possessed of an idea that they could no longer contain. Harley Farmer and I likewise. The power and the potential of the ideas that have been birthed through Harley Farmer simply could not remain unspoken any longer. We have debated them, researched them, torn them apart to ascertain their veracity, ultimately being sure enough that the potential saving of life merits taking the risk of making them public, and because seeking to bring the truth of their import to the attention of those in and with the power to transform the entire therapeutic field was falling on deaf ears and being put in front of blind eyes. Why? Well, as I wrote in 1999, in a paper entitled "Diseases of Meaning, Manifestations of Health, and Metaphor", concepts and ideas can be seen to be like micro-organisms because they can and do spread. Those with deafness and blindness need to be infected through whichever portal they will respond to, and that may mean vanity, fame and/or fortune, and the power and impact of the public voice once informed.

Look how far the ideas of Pasteur and Lister have replicated and spread, spawning vast industries, provoking vast amounts of research in the fields of microbiology, genetics and immunology, not to mention pharmacology and pharmaceuticals. All this being the result of seemingly absurd ideas that flew in the face of the known, coming from the unseen (from whence ultimately everything comes), calling for a shift in perception and meaning in the early 1800s, and requiring the courage and spirit of endeavour that arise from holding the value of human life and truth to be greater than remaining wedded to the sacred cows of prevailing paradigms of practice, politics and economics. The same is true in this extraordinary Covid-19 pandemic and the ideas expressed in *Coronoia*.

The beauty of what Harley Farmer articulates is that it requires no evocation of conspiracy to understand nor to implement. It leaves the whole world of conspiracy open to those who wish to explore and understand at ever deeper levels, and in any manner they wish, without in any way detracting from the fact that a simple application and understanding of the results of already copious extant science could radically alter, and possibly even reverse, the conditions in which the SARS-CoV-2 virus does what it has naturally evolved to do – namely to access the alveolar cells in the lungs, enter them, use the cells' resources to replicate, take over its host and spread.

So what is the sacred cow that is being so challenged here and on what basis? It is the fact that at the very least, alcohol and solvent-based sanitisers should be banned from use in clinical settings such as we find ourselves in during this pandemic. It is the fact that because alcohol and other solvents are very effective sanitisers *outside* the body, and are safe when applied *outside* the body, it is assumed that they therefore must be used to protect people in environments where they are at risk of infection – especially Covid-19. However, what that assumption fails completely to recognise is that alcohol, if inhaled or ingested, can do exactly the opposite *inside* the body, and especially the lungs, paradoxically making it easier for the virus to enter, gain access to the cells and multiply exponentially in a perfect environment to support and nourish it.

You may rightly ask why? Quite simply it is because alcohol and solvent molecules, whether in the form of vapours or within the blood following ingestion, act on the external mucus lining of the cells that is designed to protect them from the entry of viruses and other micro-organisms, so that the cells can function as they are designed to do in supporting the exchange of oxygen and carbon dioxide across their surfaces to fuel the essential life-sustaining processes of metabolism, and without which none of us can survive.

If a substance that behaves one way *outside* the body does exactly the opposite *inside* the body, rendering the person much more vulnerable to infection, even if only sniffed as a vapour, why would one use it, especially in the face of a body of evidence that at the very least deserves serious attention? Why does it continue to be the stipulated protocol promulgated by the WHO globally, when there are alternatives that have been in existence for years that are not only as effective but also much safer to use *outside* the body, especially on the skin of those having to apply the sanitisers (which will now include children all over the world) and who can react with painful dermatitis and inflammation as a result? Furthermore these alternative agents do not create mucus-dissolving vapours when inhaled and are also not only safe to apply to the skin and lead to healing, but even safe to ingest, with no deleterious effects on those same alveolar cells. Why?

This is where we find ourselves having to deal with one of the most potent aspects of what I call Diseases of Meaning. This is the hidden, unseen vector of the meanings that underpin behaviours at individual, community and governmental levels. It means too that Covid-19 and the entire situation we find ourselves in, is fundamentally a disease of meaning – scientifically in our interpretation of the data and what we believe it to mean, and in the power of our unconscious beliefs that are simultaneously driving and governing our behaviours at every level. Knowledge is one thing. Inspiring action, i.e. a change in behaviour, means addressing attitudes, beliefs and motives that can appear to be intransigent. In this situation, to listen, absorb, understand and then act requires taking in the available scientific evidence and taking on ideas that challenge accepted wisdom and practice.

It means challenging an entire industry of manufacture and supply. It means truly putting human life before politics and economics and acting on it. It means Truth being more important than expediency. It means being willing to change behaviours and protocols. It means critically evaluating the meaning of the already extant evidence and risking change even when the hallowed industry standard bearer, in this case the WHO, continues to advise otherwise. It means taking on board that for decades we may have inadvertently not only facilitated the suffering and death of millions but also unwittingly created the perfect breeding ground for the evolution of this transformed ACE-2 receptor-hugging virus.

The difference here is that we still have time to act. But we need to act fast. We can now communicate globally within seconds. So, just as the world effectively shut down within a matter of a few days early in 2020, the ideas and evidence suggested in Harley Farmer's book become a viral pandemic in their own right, only this time we actively want everyone to be infected. The idea, the message, being that swapping alcohol and solvent-based sanitisers for use against Covid-19 for quaternary ammonium compounds derived from coconut oil in 99% water, could help protect people from infection far more effectively by no longer dissolving the mucus lining of the lung cells with solvent vapours. And that applies not just in hospitals and intensive care wards. It means peoples' homes, schools, offices, transport, shops, restaurants, libraries – anywhere that people have been using alcohol and solvent-based products over recent months and years.

All that stated, we must hope and pray, i.e focus and direct our attention, as Harley Farmer exhorts us to do repeatedly in the pages of this book, so that these words will not just be read and understood but that they will be acted upon immediately and with urgency. With current evidence, and failing totally unforeseen changes to the behaviour of the virus, the situation ahead of us is very serious and the outlook potentially bleak. We do not have long. Autumn is under way in the UK and winter is coming. As Harley Farmer states in the last chapter, we could be facing over 100,000 deaths in the UK alone if we fail to act. He is not alone in quoting such figures, and they are not extreme compared to some. The science supports him. With only perhaps 6% of the population of the UK currently infected, and with the current behaviours of the population, as the weather changes and the natural seasonal infections begin to take their hold, the situation is likely to escalate exponentially, aided and abetted by current clinical practice with alcohol, which may be effectively making conditions for infection and spread ideal for the virus to thrive.

With over 35 years' experience in the medical arena, as someone deeply interested in what enables people to heal rather than being wedded to particular systems of ideas, I am certain that Covid-19 is a disease of meaning at many levels, physically, mentally and spiritually – in other words a reflection of our consciousness which we can evolve just as the virus has evolved. Therein lies our hope at all levels. Harley Farmer's *Coronoia: What the WHO failed to tell us and the UK Cabinet refused to hear* touches on all of these. It does so with a clear, evidence-based and accessible scientific foundation that brings into focus the natural phenomenon of mutation and viral evolution. It leads us naturally into asking what can sustain life and optimise immunity and vitality in the face of multiple comorbidities. Being willing to question, being willing to evaluate and being willing to shift perception and meaning will prove to be life-saving. This is what it means to be a true humanitarian dedicated to saving and optimising life, in my opinion.

Please read this book – even some of it. If Harley Farmer is correct, and there is good evidence that he is likely to be, then his hypothesis has the potential to save many millions of lives and transform many more over the generations to come. Furthermore it will help spawn new avenues of research and understanding. The key, though, is for you, the reader, to fully realise that it depends also on you, on each one of us, because currently politicians may be so busy, so preoccupied with their own rhetoric and meaning, that they fail to see and hear. Together we become a force for creative change. Together we can see that meanings matter in the guise of raw hard data, and also in the guise of emotional, psychological and spiritual beliefs and motivations. If we don't address them all, we will not be able to bring about change, the consequences of which don't bear thinking about. And the very real psycho-physical impact of the fear-mongering and draconian measures enacted to seek to control people to control the virus, combined with the vapours, only serve to weaken the immune system further. In this situation, using the ideas and measures expounded in this book, we have the potential to seriously impact our populations locally, nationally and internationally. I'm in. Are you? It brings us back to Hamlet's words with which I began – "The readiness is all." For Hamlet it also meant the readiness to die in the duel, because what had even greater meaning for him than his own potential death was his not engaging in the battle at all. We all have choices to make. I for one will be bringing this to the attention of my patients and colleagues and supporting this message whole-heartedly until it is proven otherwise. Harley Farmer's book deserves to be read and he is to be deeply thanked for his indefatigable efforts.

PREFACE

This first edition opens with what I sincerely hope will be the title of the second edition. If sufficient people help, the second half of the title will become "and what the UK Cabinet grasped immediately".

For 20 years I've been campaigning to show alcohol hand sanitisers are not serving patients well and to have alcohol hand hygiene products seen in their true light as hazardous substances. The campaign has always been based on evidence published in the peer-reviewed medical literature. It combines medical evidence with common sense derived from other aspects of human health.

The campaign is based on science, and during the Covid-19 crisis the UK Cabinet has repeatedly said they are being "guided by the science". Yet they are not hearing one relevant piece of science.

I simply ask if it is wise to positively ensure solvent vapours are present deep in the lungs of Covid-19 victims. My reading of the science suggests that could be the worst thing to do.

Covid-19 is a very fast-moving global challenge. Fast action is required with frequent changes as new details emerge. I spent months attempting to reach the Cabinet quietly. To no avail. Then I launched a new website newgenne.com to bring my reading of the science to public attention. This book shows more action was required in order to convey the science.

On that basis I present the first edition of this book suggesting the UK Cabinet refused to hear this aspect of the science. Frankly I do not care why they refused to hear. Perhaps they were just so busy they lacked time. Either way, the fact that you are reading the first edition of this book means the message has not been assimilated into action. If the Cabinet had acted in either proving or disproving my thesis that alcohol vapours were helping the virus kill people, then this book would not have been published.

In fast-moving situations like Covid-19, it is to be expected that many single-focused suggestions will be inappropriate and rightly cast aside after due examination by those with personal responsibility for the safety of the UK population. That may be the outcome awaiting this book. If so, I will have achieved my first objective of having the science I present considered and debated.

If the science in this text is valid and appropriate, yet the Cabinet and their medical advisors choose to ignore that science, then very serious questions will be asked. Others are better qualified than me to pursue those questions as legal action would be the obvious outcome. Those questions should be asked and anyone who needs to be held to account for needless deaths should be dealt with by the full force of the law. That is retrospective action.

My chosen role will remain one of preventing future needless deaths. That is what my decades of work has achieved, and I intend to continue in that light.

I therefore end this preface with a challenge to the reader. Can you help bring this science and its relevance to the attention of the UK Cabinet? If you can, please do so. If I'm wrong in my perspective of the science I will return to improving my thesis. If I'm right, ask yourself how you will feel if you could have acted and you are seeing ever more people dying from Covid-19 while they are breathing in solvent vapours.

This challenge is deliberately offered to the public. The UK Cabinet are busy and they need our help.

Any politician in opposition parties who chooses to use this text to attack the Government will be invited to disclose what they have done to remove the solvent alcohol vapours from hospitals in their constituency. This is above party politics. On the day I am writing this preface, over 40,000 people have died in the UK after testing positive for SARS-CoV-2 infection within 28 days prior to their death.

I implore you to do the right thing and join in the battle to prevent that number becoming just a drop in the ocean. At the moment, the UK population is still naive to this virus as relatively few people have actually been infected. The disaster we witnessed in the first half of 2020 will pale into insignificance if the second calamity I and many others are predicting happens in the winter of 2020 to 2021. I fear we may look back on 2020 as the gentle Covid-19 year compared to 2021.

Please do what you can to have the second edition of this book published with the title:

Coronoia®: What the WHO failed to tell us and the UK Cabinet grasped immediately.

Thank you.

Dr Harley Farmer PhD BVSc(hons) BVBiol(path) MRCVS
CEO NewGenne Ltd
26 August 2020

CHAPTER 1

In recognition of anticipated comments, I begin by stressing that the Dr before my name relates to me having a PhD. Please read this work in full and clear recognition that I am a Doctor of Philosophy. I have no medical qualifications, which ironically makes me more qualified to present the thesis on which this book is based. I care about the *individual* who I feel is not being served well by the establishment. I find questions, create others and encompass the skills of many like-minded people as, collectively, we seek to establish answers.

This is being written in August 2020 in the midst of an unprecedented global pandemic. Specific questions are asked and equally specific answers and interpretations are provided. The Covid-19 pandemic is rapidly evolving and this book can only include what is known now and what can be reasonably surmised of the future.

Key questions include:

- Where did the virus come from?
- Why did we not see it coming?
- What is the key factor favouring the virus?
- How did it manage to spread so quickly?
- Why is the death rate following infection so high?
- Where will the virus strike next?
- Will we all be safe when a vaccine arrives?

Other topics will include what a virus is, how the Covid-19 virus attacks cells, how new virus particles are made and why viruses change.

The best starting place is to suggest why your time spent reading this book in its entirety will be time well invested. My experience has centred on preventing infections by microbes like viruses and bacteria. In my professional view the best way to prevent infections is to keep the number of microbes below the number needed for infection to occur. In the context of Covid-19, that includes reducing the number of virus particles made and released by each infected person. Other aspects like killing virus particles and preventing their spread between people are important to me too. Fortunately many other people are providing their expertise on such aspects, whereas I am usually alone in ensuring fewer virus particles are made in the first place.

To me, the best way to have fewer Covid infections is to have fewer coronavirus particles present to do the infecting. Reduce the number made and you reduce the number present and able to infect.

I'm best known for preventing Norovirus outbreaks. That virus has been known by many names including the winter vomiting virus, vomiting and diarrhoea virus and cruise ship virus. It's considered by many virus experts to be the most infectious virus known to infect humans. Very few virus particles are needed to establish an infection. It is also a very hard virus to kill with disinfectants.

The Covid-19 virus is far easier to address than Norovirus. It's easier to inactivate with disinfectants and its spread between people is easier to prevent. I therefore offer the view that since I have so many years of success in halting Norovirus, I will have useful ideas to suggest in halting the Covid-19 virus.

If you want a way of validating that, ask yourself if Norovirus outbreaks are common in UK hospitals, schools and care homes. If you are from another nation consider your local situation. Since such outbreaks are so common despite the best efforts of the government infection prevention authorities, consider whether you want something new to compare with advice those authorities are providing on how to stop this new virus from spreading.

The Covid-19 virus has spread in an alarming manner. Yet the health authorities from the World Health Organisation (WHO) downwards had their best prevention principles and procedures in place before the new virus was even recognised. Those principles and procedures failed to stop the spread. I will present science-based evidence that allows me to ask if those principles and procedures are likely to have *enhanced the spread*.

Since this is a book intended to be read by the general public as well as medical experts, I would like to say at this early stage that you will find a complete absence of conspiracy theories. When you see the sequence of events presented I hope you will agree with me that no conspiracy theories are needed to explain what has happened. It is all logical and it all follows the long-established laws of Nature.

Conspiracy theories have their place as they can sometimes point to facets of a story that warrant serious scientific investigation. The value of "an old wives tale" can be immense. Personally I love using conspiracy theories in the novels I write. This book is non-fiction; it is based on facts and the content is real. You will see I present the appropriate references to articles from peer-reviewed medical journals to ensure readers can remain confident throughout. When you see a number in brackets after a statement, for example (Reference 5), that number refers to the reference presented in the bibliography at the end of the book. I have strenuously avoided using too many technical references, restricting myself to just the number required to allow confidence of credibility in what is presented.

The only area of conjecture is how I choose to weave the proven facts into the Covid-19 virus narrative. If this book generates the amount of collaboration and support that I hope will arise, it's perfectly possible that the second edition will follow within a matter of months.

I am relying on challenges from my scientific and medical colleagues. Those who just want to shut down the debate are likely to be left behind in this fast-moving topic. There will be many more who see places where they can strengthen the thesis I offer. Those colleagues may become the leaders in the debate while I settle back into the shadows to continue my preference for deep thinking. It's all changing so rapidly, any predictions made by anyone must be speculation.

This pandemic has taken humanity by surprise. The word unprecedented is justified. Team effort will become our best defence and the greatest number of team players will come from the general public. There is nothing mysterious about this supposedly new virus. It is following the laws of Nature. I will suggest it is the actions of humans which advanced a virus in balance with its host into a pandemic virus killing untold numbers of its host.

The virus has no psyche. It lacks an agenda. I will explain why a virus particle made of proteins and genetic material is given a colloquial persona and why it can be useful to utilise the persona. Given the choice between saying:

- the virus spread or
- we spread the virus

the former is less challenging to humanity's ego. We can then blame the virus rather than people. It is playing with words, and when people are this scared that can be very helpful as long as you acknowledge what you are doing and explain why. I intend this book to be inclusive as all the readers will be humans and this virus is attacking humanity. After we have all beaten the virus some of us will turn the collective effort into division. I await their post-apocalyptic synopsis with open glee.

Until then, I ask your permission to be inclusive while I do what little I can to bring all of humanity on a journey of factual reality. You already know how scary the Covid-19 story has been so far. I intend to show you how much worse it will become if we fail to utilise the available choices.

CHAPTER 2

I recall the image on television of a reporter standing in the centre of a wide street in Wuhan, China. The street should have been filled with cars. Yet it was empty.

Something of great magnitude had occurred in Wuhan. Something *invisible* to the human eye had caused that *visible* image. To be more correct, the *effect* of that invisible something had caused humans to remove their cars.

The effect was fear.

That same fear removed the cars from streets in one city after another around the world.

National economies went into lockdown. An invisible entity was controlling humanity.

What do humans feel when they are that far out of control? Paranoia. It would be foolish to feel otherwise. To do so would be complete denial. So paranoia prevailed.

A new coronavirus had arrived. A new phenomenon arose when coronavirus met paranoia. What appears when you join the words coronavirus and paranoia and shorten it?

Coronoia.

The consequences of that global fear are all too apparent.

The "invisible enemy", as some national leaders tend to call it, had arrived and humans were pushed into submission. Or to be more correct, humans *chose* submission.

Humans did the best they could with the resources they had available at the time. One of their choices was Coronoia. I ask if those in charge had chosen to completely ignore another available choice. It's my view they did, and the medical experts we trust to guide us have a long history of ignoring that specific choice.

The purpose of this book is to guide national governments to their own realisations that another choice was available, is still available and it is very easy to implement.

If humanity continues to do what it did in the first half of 2020 it can expect to achieve the same in the second half. Unfortunately the death rate is expected to be far greater in the second half. I will present my views on why that appalling statistic is awaiting us and share some estimates of how many new deaths are being discussed.

The collective wisdom of those advising humanity led to Coronoia. That collective wisdom chose to ignore one resource. I will explain how that occurrence, which failed to serve us well, could happen. The outcome was inevitable. I will also do my best to help the general public guide those in power who utilised that limited collective wisdom. The medical experts did their best and hundreds of thousands of people died of Covid-19.

Something more is needed if we want to prevent far more from dying. The something is a change in mindset. If you want to achieve something different it's best to do something different. Coronoia is an uncomfortable feeling. It signifies that we are losing, and unless there is change we will continue to lose against the "invisible enemy". That name signifies a negative mindset with all the hallmarks of becoming a self-fulfilling prophecy. We are akin to the rabbit compelled to remain stationary by the car headlights. The rabbit would be served well by a little momentum.

Yet I believe it will require momentum from the public to have governments incorporate the missing choice into our battle against this new coronavirus. Momentum is calculated by multiplying velocity by mass. It's rare for the general public to provide much velocity, whereas it always delivers a lot of mass. A tiny amount of velocity multiplied by a lot of mass equals huge momentum. Just what we want.

All the public need do is consider my thesis presented in this book and decide whether it is logical and holds true to their values. Should they choose to agree, that simple act provides a tiny amount of velocity as the view of society will have moved. Each person will have done their part to help humanity overcome Coronoia.

Obviously should any individuals take it upon themselves to join vocal and very public demonstrations outside government buildings, that will add to their contribution of velocity. A pleasing number of individuals will take that extra action which means I can concentrate on performing my preferred role, removing from me any need to push anyone into action. I can, and will, leave the choice to each individual.

My role is to get the thinkers thinking so the talkers have something new to talk about. I will avoid anything akin to telling people what to do. If some choose to do nothing despite my efforts, that is the right decision for them at the time. If others choose to do far more than I envisage, then again it's the right decision for them at the time. Humanity will be served better by the second group so my hope is for this book to embolden the action takers.

The Covid-19 coronavirus took humanity by surprise and we know to our massive cost that the actions taken by those of influence failed to serve us well. The infection spread rapidly around the world so our initial focus is best directed at the principles of infection prevention.

This book presents a positive suggestion. The best way to prove that is to explain the reality of infection prevention as it has been allowed to prevail over recent generations. Sadly that history has been one of repeated failure to stop microbes killing people. Tens of thousands of people die every year from avoidable healthcare associated infections around the developed world when the best and most current infection prevention principles are being used. When a new and deadly coronavirus appeared it was inevitable that many deaths would follow if those same principles were used as our best effort to stop the virus. If the favoured principles could not prevent deaths from common bacteria we know how to defeat, how would those same principles stop a virus we had never encountered before? They wouldn't and they didn't.

Failed infection prevention principles had become the accepted global "gold standard" before this virus showed itself in Wuhan. We know those failed principles did not stop it. Even worse, I intend to demonstrate why those principles favoured the virus by enhancing its spread and increasing the likelihood that it would kill more of the people it infected than was necessary.

CHAPTER 3

It is true that no-one saw this virus coming. At first it had no name so medical protocol meant we had to wait for the appropriate authorities to give it an official name. They chose SARS-CoV-2. In marketing terms it's far from a catchy name which is why the general public prefer to keep calling it coronavirus. In contrast, to those of us who value the thinking of the naming group, it means a great deal. That of course will not stop me calling it the Covid-19 virus and the coronavirus in this text. Even I find SARS-CoV-2 an encumbrance.

It is not a new virus in the view of the experts; it's the original SARS virus with just enough changes for them to say it's version 2 rather than the same virus coming around again. It has simply changed a bit.

Suddenly the mystique has gone. It's the same virus that has effectively hidden itself since its first appearance in 2003 until it surfaced again in 2019 with a few changes.

It will have been following some form of laws in that time. Since humans did not know it was coming it wasn't following our laws. That means it will have been following the laws of Nature. Further mystique is removed as we know a lot about the laws of Nature. We know what a lot of other viruses have done under those laws which allows us to begin seeking clues.

Since I am writing this in August 2020 I have the advantage of hindsight. I can begin to know where I should look for its tracks. We all know it appeared, killed, spread and as it did so national economies were devastated. The missing clues will be found by looking at what it was doing before it appeared in Wuhan.

This SARS-CoV-2 virus, like all other viruses, is just a collection of chemical molecules. It's a unique blend of proteins and genetic material, which for this virus is RNA. A virus cannot replicate itself as it lacks the biological equipment required. A virus is far smaller than a living cell so it gains entry into a cell and causes the cell to make more viruses using the cell's biological equipment. To do that the virus must have a way of overcoming the natural defences of the target cell.

The virus lacks a mind, it has no psyche, no agenda. It cannot tell humans what to do. Yet it will take advantage of any opportunity created by humans. Just as water will spread to fill a hole we have made, this virus spread with remarkable ease. First within people, then between people, then between nations. Continuing the water analogy, the virus needed humans to do something which allowed it to spread at that rate.

This coronavirus has always been easy to kill with common disinfectants that were extensively used before, during and after version 2 of the virus was discovered. Yet it still spread alarmingly quickly and easily despite our best chemical defences. What if our infection prevention principles made it easier for the virus to spread and kill so many people? What if our primary defence for other viruses was our greatest weakness against this virus? What if this virus had, during its shadow years between 2003 and 2019, been quietly adapting to take advantage of that weakness? All three questions will be answered in subsequent chapters.

The challenge is to determine what humans did that so favoured an inanimate virus. Water is inanimate yet tsunamis are well known when water is pushed by a physical effect like an earthquake. The water / virus analogy allows me to ask what led to the virus spreading. Was it pushed or did an absence of a natural barrier allow it to flow?

CHAPTER 4

The WHO has a blind spot. It's inevitable as every organisation has blind spots. For all its many virtues the WHO is an amalgam, a committee of global proportion. All their experts correctly share their life's experiences and knowledge, and humanity has gained benefits from that generosity on many occasions. I favour the WHO and will do all I can to support it. However, in global terms I am just one person who has spent decades trying to have the WHO consider that it has a blind spot. Needless to say when it was focusing on various flu viruses and Ebola, it had little time to sit with me while I explained my different ideas.

Then a strain of virus appeared that had effectively slotted straight into what I had long been calling the WHO's blind spot. By definition they will not have seen it coming as they were blind to it.

In such a large organisation, only people who share the collective's perspective tend to remain in the collective. It's a law of Nature which encompasses all living things, including humans. History teaches what happens when human collectives consistently ignore one obvious fact. Nature will concoct something that will take advantage. Humans will find themselves outsmarted and need to play catch-up. Covid-19 is precisely that.

The virus adapted itself to the blind spot over many years and we only noticed after it had taken full advantage and gained a firm hold. What humanity considered to be one of its greatest defences gave the virus its greatest advantage.

A blind spot serves few people well. When it involves all of humanity we suddenly have an absolutely huge resource at our disposal. Rather than harping back to what the WHO failed to see or tell us, we can ask what each of us is going to do so the WHO can help us all catch up and eventually win.

Even though I do not work *for* the WHO I consider myself to work *with* the organisation. When they did not need my help I was content to develop my ideas. Even now they are likely to feel they are too busy to seek my help and I'm relaxed if that is how they feel. They are indeed very busy so I prefer to let them proceed as only they can.

While that is happening, I have the opportunity to muster immense human resources to best help the WHO help humanity. It sounds very grand, yet what it really translates to is many people sharing their experiences and views. Mine relate to having overcome other viruses over many years. My contribution lies in knowing how to balance the existence of a virus with the absence of illness. Other people will have equally useful experiences and together we will win.

Nobody dies just because they were infected with this Covid virus. They only die if the virus gets the upper hand against the person's lungs and immune system. The virus needs a lot more than just access to one human cell. It needs something that favours the virus, and that something, as prescribed by the laws of Nature, could easily relate to a blind spot that has been in place for many decades, long before the original SARS virus left bats and entered humans.

When new microbes appear it's logical and correct for routine long-established defences to be utilised. It's normal for weaknesses in the defence system to become obvious and exposed during challenges. Even more so when the weakness magnifies the threat. When that happens, experts can become overwhelmed, making it harder for them to realise they have other choices. Even more so if the obvious choice means dismantling one of the main defences they have relied upon their entire working lives.

I have a life-long history of wondering about the establishment. Very early in my life it was made obvious how poorly the establishment viewed my repeated questions. If you want more detail I refer you to the dr-harley.com website which I use as my author's public face.

My questioning skills began with how my society was treating the indigenous Aboriginals in central Australia over 50 years ago. I was told to remain quiet as it was unlikely a child in grade three would know the full story. Only many years later was the "lost generation" revealed, exposing an uncomfortable aspect of Australia's history. It turned out my questions were a bit too close to the truth. I now appreciate the establishment at the time had a justification for its actions, and only time and hindsight showed how one-sided that justification was.

I subsequently studied psychology and learned the value of finding and sharing choices. Given the predominant position we choose to give the WHO, its experts have an obligation to seek out and utilise all the available choices.

History will show the WHO experts showed all the signs of believing their combined experience would be the only way to control the spread of the Covid coronavirus. History shows they would have been able to better serve us all if they had one more choice. This book is intended to be part of that history.

CHAPTER 5

Certain nations can be seen as having been more successful against Covid-19. In the spring of 2020 the number of deaths in China seemed devastatingly high. Several months later, having lost just 3,000 people seems amazingly successful. Covid-19 is forcing us to realign our perspectives.

What did the European governments choose to do differently from those in the western Pacific region? Or was it something they chose to not do as well?

Even the Republic of Korea (South Korea) can gain from having more choices. I speak as one who played a part in halting their MERS coronavirus outbreak several years ago. My company air-freighted tonnes of hand sanitiser from the UK to the ROK during MERS. My hand sanitiser was free of alcohol, as it had been since 2000. The positive contribution it made was proportionate to the amount used in comparison to others.

The MERS outbreak forced the Republic of Korea to become hyper-aware which put them at an advantage when Covid-19 arrived.

For me, the main gain from their MERS episode was a question I was able to frame from half a world away. Why did people continue dying from MERS in one of their best hospitals long after they stopped dying elsewhere? It looked to me as though humans were doing something that favoured the virus. Like all coronaviruses, the MERS virus was comparatively easy to inactivate with standard disinfectants. Since the most widely respected hospital in Seoul had access to the best and most powerful disinfectants, could it have been one of those that favoured the virus and maintained the deaths?

For many reasons my main focus was on solvent vapours from disinfectants, both those used on floors and surfaces and also alcohol hand sanitisers. MERS enters cells by a different receptor than the one used by SARS and SARS-2. Yet there was one fundamental aspect they had in common, and Covid-19 allowed me to test my question.

History is a good teacher if you are prepared to learn and test. When the Diamond Princess cruise ship was moored in Yokohama harbour because a few people on board were positive for coronavirus, it should have been an ideal quarantine facility. I tried to communicate with the owners of the Diamond Princess citing the fact that I had once been on a relevant committee of the cruise industry when I was helping them combat Norovirus. I received no response from the cruise company, which left me as a witness.

As anticipated, the Covid virus spread rapidly despite the common and widespread use of alcohol hand sanitisers, the cruise industry's main defence against infections. Ironically that industry knew alcohol sanitisers did not stop Norovirus and they were only used because their passengers expected to have them. That meant the passengers on the Diamond Princess would have had ample alcohol sanitiser. My question was whether the solvent vapours rising from warm hands treated with the liquid alcohol were playing a role in transmission of the coronavirus. Since I was not provided the opportunity to help, I could only watch as a knowledgeable bystander.

History shows what happened on the Diamond Princess. It became such a disaster that national governments began repatriating their citizens. Rather than being an ideal quarantine facility, the ship had become a smouldering pot of infection transmission. The important point is that the alcohol placed on hands would have inactivated any coronavirus it encountered on hands. However, it was the solvent vapours I was interested in, something the cruise line declined to let me share with them.

When something similar happened in northern Italy and then Spain, I had no route to share my technical point. However, when Covid-19 exploded in the UK, I had ample ways of attempting to share. I received absolutely no acknowledgement from the UK Government. The local Member of Parliament for where I live did pass my idea to the health authorities and they chose to make no contact. The local Member of Parliament for where my company is situated did not even acknowledge my emails. That person is a Secretary of State so the absence of any response was telling.

Therefore I have been forced to be a bystander while people around me are dying and my business colleagues are seeing their companies crippled by the shutdown.

The only reason this book is being written rests on the fact that I have failed completely in my attempt to convey my thesis quietly to those who would most benefit from my technical expertise. Please keep in mind that the UK health authorities know that facilities using our products do not have Norovirus outbreaks, so those same authorities will have known we had expertise in combatting viruses. The only reason I'm relaxed about being ignored to that extent is because all those tens of thousands of Covid deaths and the massive national debt are the Government's primary concern rather than mine. The UK Cabinet chose to keep that to themselves by not taking heed of the wealth of useful information available within the UK. It had nothing to do with me personally as I knew other useful people who had been ignored too.

I also knew that if the UK Cabinet chose to not listen, I had the option of writing another book and using that to generate interest in the UK public. I am just one person among 65 million. If the number of people interested in my thesis was raised sufficiently high, there is an increased chance the UK Cabinet will listen and come to their own realisation that they have at least one more choice.

Since I've been on this sort of theme for over 20 years I appreciate how unlikely it is that the UK Cabinet will listen, let alone take appropriate action. They have chosen their path and over 40,000 people have died within 28 days of testing positive for the Covid-19 virus.

Nobody can know how many would have died if alcohol vapours were not in the air they breathed in. Equally nobody can know how many died *because* that solvent vapour was in their air.

My purpose now is to alert the public to what has happened and make it very clear that the UK Cabinet has so far refused to hear. I see my role as helping in any way I can to guide the UK Cabinet to their own realisation that a choice, which the WHO failed to tell us exists, is readily available to the Cabinet members. There is little to be gained in me raising my voice. Far more will be achieved by having many UK citizens enter the debate. If anyone in the UK Cabinet chooses to feel embarrassed by our revelations that will simply mean I have more work to do in helping them reach their own realisation. As I mentioned in the preface, I would be delighted to have the second edition of this book carry a subtitle saying "What the WHO failed to tell us and the UK Cabinet grasped immediately".

However, I sense that will only happen if the UK public become alerted to what is being done in their name. If they can see that, one very minor change could remove something that I believe is favouring the virus.

CHAPTER 6

This is the appropriate point to introduce my thesis. Since we are in such a rapidly evolving situation, I have chosen to extract the following text from my website newgenne.com along with the date of provenance. This version was written and posted in July and a lot has happened since. If you want to follow the sequential changes, please keep close watch on the website as that is where the updated versions will be presented.

The following text is a straight extract from the website taken on 9 August 2020 under the Covid-19 button. The extract ends at the end of this chapter.

Thesis on how SARS-CoV-2 arose

This is an evolving thesis which will evolve further as Covid-19 evolves.

In nature when a new virus gains entry to a new host there may be significant deaths in the host species. Things usually settle down and the virus finds a way of co-existing with the host so the mortality rate falls. The virus will still be replicated without the host being killed and a form of subtle parasitism develops. That is Nature's way and in many cases the new virus becomes part of the host biome with only specialist virologists and medical historians having any reason to consider the virus which has now concealed itself.

In late 2002 a novel coronavirus caused Severe Acute Respiratory Syndrome (SARS), a new human disease with an alarmingly high mortality rate. The severity and rapid spread induced strong international collaboration and the virus which came from bats via civet cats to humans was called SARS-CoV. The virus attacked Alveolar Type II cells (AT2 cells) in alveoli, the tiny air sacs deep within our lungs. To do so, it first attached to the ACE2 receptors on the airway facing side of the AT2 cells. Those receptors are protected by a mucus called pulmonary surfactant which is produced by the AT2 cells.

The SARS epidemic faded and the world moved on with little apparent concern for whether the virus had become established in humans.

If the SARS virus was to become concealed in humans it makes sense for it to be predominantly in people where it could gain the most access to its target receptor. That would require people with less effective pulmonary surfactant, the covering which normally defends the ACE2 receptor on the virus' target AT2 cells.

The human group which suits that definition best is the elderly. Advanced age is known to reduce pulmonary surfactant integrity. For the balances of nature to be maintained the virus would not cause mortality in its new host sub-group. It would infect sufficient cells for enough virus particles to be breathed out to infect sufficient new people, all without overt mortality.

In late 2019, long after SARS disappeared, a new coronavirus arose and because of its close similarity to the SARS virus it was named SARS-CoV-2. This new virus rapidly became associated with a global pandemic of greater magnitude than SARS with many more deaths.

Both viruses gain entry by attaching to the ACE2 receptors on AT2 cells deep within the lungs.

The key differences in the two coronaviruses relate to the proteins on the ends of the viral spikes. The more recent virus has a much tighter fit with the receptor and it has a new way of arranging its spike proteins to more effectively evade the immune system. The information currently available induces me to view the newer virus as being the original virus which has developed two significant protein changes.

How did the virus remain concealed for seventeen years while it adapted so well to the target receptors on the host lung cells? Perhaps its effect was being masked by a common condition of the elderly; one that ends many lives every day.

Elderly people often die of bacterial pneumonia. A virus subtly lurking in the lungs could easily and justifiably be missed if the deceased person had the usual array of bacteria. Common things occur commonly and clinicians assisting patients in terminal decline should be concentrating on their patients rather than looking for the unknown.

The normal reduction in integrity of the pulmonary surfactant produced by the AT2 cells in the elderly means the innate defences of the mucus covering the AT2 cells is progressively weakened. That would have given the coronavirus more opportunities to attach to the ACE2 receptor and progressively adapt its spike proteins to better fit the receptor.

As the virus adapted it will have infected more AT2 cells leaving less of those cells to make pulmonary surfactant resulting in less protection of the ACE2 receptors on other AT2 cells.

The combination of less effective innate protection because the elderly produced less effective surfactant and the new fact that less of the surfactant was being produced because there were fewer AT2 cells would have allowed the virus to multiply in greater numbers.

In due course doctors treating normal pneumonia in their elderly patients will have noticed slight differences in the symptoms they expected of the elderly with pneumonia.

Such changes would have initially been very subtle. Over time the patients in whom the adapted virus was gaining a hold will have been exhaling progressively more adapted virus.

The city where the new symptoms would probably be noticed first would be one where the doctors had extensive experience of SARS and the local laboratory was the world leader in bat viruses. Wuhan, in central China. They would be the most likely to recognise that the steady change was beginning to look like the original SARS.

Their proper reaction would have been to enhance best practice in infection control which meant the use of more alcohol hand sanitisers. The vapour from those alcohol products will have been breathed in by the elderly patients. Alcohol vapour dissolves the major component of pulmonary surfactant so vapour from the alcohol sanitisers would have reduced even further the surfactant protection over any remaining ACE2 receptors leading to the infection of more AT2 cells reducing even further the amount of pulmonary surfactant produced.

Patients in that situation would have begun showing symptoms even more reminiscent of SARS.

On the basis of that very frightening development the hospital teams should have intensified the use of best practice and used even more alcohol hand sanitisers. They will have been seeking the protective effect of the liquid alcohol on hands with no reason to wonder if the vapour arising from the warm hands was exacerbating the demise of their patients.

I suggest SARS-CoV slowly adapted over seventeen years and had settled into the subtle parasitic balance expected under the laws of Nature. That avoids the need to explain where a new virus arose, as new viruses are very rare. An existing virus which adapted to its host is easier to explain.

As the new SARS-like disease killed more elderly people, medical staff will have been sufficiently scared for their own lives that they used more and more alcohol sanitisers delivering more and more alcohol vapour to the already infected cells deep in the lung alveoli.

SARS-CoV, the original virus, caused a disturbing number of deaths and the disease it caused was rapidly restricted. Nature's rules meant SARS-CoV-2 was in balance with its host and there is no logical reason for it to suddenly kill hundreds of thousands of people. Something that was not in tune with Nature's usual rules was involved. Mankind's trait of having solvent vapours enter deep into the lungs of patients is certainly artificial and beyond Nature's boundaries.

Did alcohol vapour, an ignored byproduct of a chemical used on hands, artificially tip balance into pandemic?

Alcohol vapour is known to enter the lungs of people using alcohol hand sanitisers. The vapour simply passed into the blood or was breathed out again. There was little or no attention paid to whether it was affecting the integrity of the pulmonary surfactant. The progressive adaptation of a virus to one specific receptor changed that.

Now the vapour was further damaging already impaired surfactant which will have been to the benefit of the adapted coronavirus.

For seventeen years the virus had remained concealed in common bacterial pneumonia so nobody will have had reason to search for it. Only when signs caused by the virus became apparent among the normal signs of terminal pneumonia would any clinician have had reason to wonder. By then the new signs were looking reminiscent of SARS so the correct reaction of the hospital staff will have been to use more alcohol sanitisers. For all previous diseases that was the best reaction as prescribed by the World Health Organisation.

For Covid-19 it may have been the worst possible thing to do.

What now?

Until this thesis is proven wrong it would be extremely unwise to continue subjecting patients infected with SARS-CoV-2 to alcohol vapours. Alcohol hand sanitisers in Covid-19 wards should be replaced immediately with effective alternative products that do not release solvent vapours. Such products are readily available.

Failure to do so will leave the medical authorities with the need to refute my thesis if more patients die from Covid-19. Since thousands are expected to die in the coming months this is especially pertinent.

Should I be proven wrong I'll work on adapting my thesis. If I am not proven wrong, either because the authorities chose not to bother trying or I am proven at least partially correct, I will continue to champion one question.

Are alcohol hand sanitisers playing a significant role in Covid-19 deaths?

If so, the SARS-CoV-2 virus was in balance with its host, even if that balance was turning gradually in favour of the virus in elderly dying people. It was the use of alcohol hand sanitisers which turned balance into pandemic. Continued use will continue the pandemic.

The virus will remain as something humanity lives with. The virus/alcohol combination may be something many people die with.

Could it be that Nature took the virus into balance and alcohol vapours took the virus into pandemic?

Was it balance slowly over many years and pandemic suddenly in a few months?

An obvious human response will be to apportion blame. My preference is to avoid judgement and seek inclusion. As with the SARS crisis, now is a good time to unite against one adversary. Many conspiracy theories abound and each presents plausible points. I prefer to find a sequence which fits the well-established laws of Nature. If such a sequence is plausible to the point of looking obvious, the need for conspiracy theories diminishes.

Over the many years between SARS and Covid-19 everyone did what they should have done in accordance with best practice and they followed the most appropriate scientific evidence:

- The world came together to end SARS.
- Doctors helping elderly patients dying from typical bacterial pneumonia did their job.
- When different symptoms arose in some of those patients medical teams followed established global best practice in using more alcohol hand sanitisers.
- Authorities in Wuhan recognised those new symptoms and took appropriate action.
- Other nations acted accordingly with the resources available to them at the time.

The only glaring mistake was to ignore the vapour rising from alcohol sanitisers on hands. Those products were used because the liquid alcohol, often in gel form, was the antimicrobial active. The focus was on the hands. The vapour was never part of anyone's infection prevention process and had this virus not adapted in the way it has, the vapour would still be ignored.

I prefer that no blame be apportioned in the sequence presented above.

However, from the day this document enters the public domain and alcohol vapour is known to be favouring the virus leading to more Covid-19 deaths, then blame can and should be apportioned to anyone who fails to replace the alcohol sanitisers with alternatives that do not release solvent vapours. Those non-alcohol products have been used around the world for decades. My company has one and I can refer people to others.

There are thousands of lives at risk and it is all happening in full public view. This would be a very bad time to continue supporting the use of a product which generated a side effect that contributes to thousands of deaths.

Now is one of those times to work together. The SARS virus did not go away, just as authorities are saying the Covid-19 virus will not go away. If the second virus really is the first virus in a form better adapted to reduced pulmonary surfactant integrity, it already has an excellent hold in one sector of the human population.

Continuing to favour the virus by continuing to use alcohol hand sanitisers will be ignoring the science.

Collective action to remove alcohol vapours from the Covid-19 setting is essential.
Dr Harley Farmer PhD BVSc(hons) BVBiol(path) MRCVS
CEO NewGenne Ltd newgenn.com +44 (0) 7876 747700
26 July 2020

CHAPTER 7

If the virus is just a collection of chemicals without life or any form of intelligence, how can it adapt? That is a good fundamental question that was often asked way back when humans first became capable of working on viruses. For many decades controversy raged among the scientists, with many feeling they had no reason to believe something they could not see was capable of replication. The doubters accepted bacteria as they could see them dividing by looking down a bench microscope. Viruses posed more of a challenge to the imagination.

Society still has its doubters when it comes to viruses. This coronavirus seems to fuel the doubt given how many people are asymptomatic. Those individuals never feel ill, yet an antibody test, which they also lack the technical knowledge to understand, gives a result telling them they have been infected by the virus. In times of immense trouble like those we are encountering, it is wise to allow the doubters freedom of expression. The scientists who claim to know a huge amount about viruses obviously have insufficient control to prevent the spread, and that engenders very little confidence among people who choose to doubt the very existence of the virus.

Fortunately most people in these troubled times accept the existence of artificial intelligence because it is a part of their everyday lives. I therefore use the processes of artificial intelligence as an analogy for viruses. In artificial intelligence we utilise a piece of software, a sequence of inanimate code, to perform a task. That sequence of code has no life and no intelligence. Nothing happens when the code is simply sitting there inactive. It is also important to keep in mind that the sequence of code exists in a computer of some kind. It is a sequence of digits limited to either 0 or 1. Ironically that software code is even more difficult to believe because it has only two digits.

We set that piece of software code on a task and have it do the task time and time again knowing there is a capacity within the code, amongst the 0 and 1 digits, to allow minor changes each time the task is performed. Some of those changes make the next attempt at the task less likely to succeed, and those changes don't proceed. Other changes take the code one tiny step closer to achieving the task, and those changes go forward to the next stage. The next attempt at the task is done by the code with the additional benefit of that newest tiny change in code. If the coding is correct and the task is actually achievable, the code will keep changing until it achieves the task.

Keep in mind that this intelligence, as we choose to call it, can only show itself within a computer, within hardware that provides the systems and mechanism for the code to show its intelligence. The software code is not hardware. The two are distinct and what we call artificial intelligence can only happen when the two are allowed to work together.

The next step is to introduce into the discussion the concept of computer viruses. In that case a piece of software code can infect and take over the functions of a computer. Initially it might be just one laptop. If that laptop is connected to many others via the internet, the computer virus can spread. This analogy works best when you then ask why do only some of the other laptops on the internet become infected? It's because the infected laptops had the least protection. They became infected because there was a way in and the computer virus, the piece of code, utilised it. The newly infected laptop then makes more copies of the virus which are released to infect any other laptops that lack the defences needed to keep it out.

The computer sector was wise to select the word virus for this aggressive piece of computer code. The analogy is excellent.

Most people have seen the graphics of the coronavirus on television and therefore know each virus particle has spikes on its outside. At the outer end of those spikes are three proteins arranged in a specific shape. That shape acts as a key. On the outside of the target cell which the virus wants to gain entry into are receptors which are analogous to a lock. If the key fits the lock sufficiently well the virus can gain entry. When it is inside the cell the virus has the ability to take over the production processes of the cell, processes the virus was too small to carry on its own. The genetic code within the virus is read by the cell's normal production systems and the code tells the cell to make more virus particles. That includes copies of the virus genetic material and copies of the proteins. When those are combined into a new virus particle the latter is released from the cell. When the key of the new virus particle meets the lock on another cell, it gains entry to that cell, and the newly infected cell makes more virus particles which are in turn shed from that cell, and so on.

The genetic code of the Covid-19 virus is of a type that tends to make small mistakes each time an infected cell's processes read it to make new virus particles. Some of those changes are detrimental and any particle carrying that slightly adapted code will not be replicated. In contrast, if the minor change favours the intention of the virus by making it more likely to gain entry to another cell, the change is accepted and that virus particle utilises its advantage. Subsequent copies of the virus carry that new minor adaptation.

Anything that reduces the next cell's protection will make it easier for the virus to gain entry and in time adapt, making it even easier for subsequent virus particles to have themselves replicated and released.

The changes each time are incredibly tiny. However, within the lungs of one infected person there are millions of cells and each infected cell will make an unfortunately high number of new virus particles. Among those new virus particles could be some with a new and slightly advantageous adaptation. Whether the newest virus is breathed out to infect another person, or simply gains entry to the lung cell beside the one that made it, is of vital importance to the person infected.

In my thesis, the original SARS virus initially came from bats. It then gained entry to civet cats with the inevitable small changes such a jump from one species to another would involve. From the cats it moved to humans requiring even more minor changes. Scientists could tell it was the same bat virus with minor changes. That virus's key had an adequate fit to the lock on a human lung cell for it to gain entry, be replicated and spread. The SARS epidemic which so terrified humanity was the result.

From the human perspective, the chance advantage taken by the bat virus was the opportunity to infect and adapt within civet cats. The original bat virus on its own never infected human cells, or if it did the effect was so minor nobody noticed.

In the sequence from bats to humans, the SARS virus was favoured by a step within civet cats. There was no actual intelligence in the form of intention. An opportunity was presented and among the millions and millions of virus particles made during the sequence, some developed the capacity to infect humans so severely that the humans developed a Sudden Acute Respiratory Syndrome – SARS – in sufficient numbers that humanity noticed.

It's a sequential biochemical process making the next small change to the virus's advantage. It's a chance event with only favourable adaptations being carried forward to the next generation of the virus. The only laws followed would be the laws of Nature.

CHAPTER 8

The original SARS coronavirus had between late-2002 and 2019 to make sequential adaptations until it became SARS-2. It had ample humans to replicate in, and within each infected human there were huge numbers of its target lung cells. In this numbers game there were ample opportunities for an RNA virus to undergo numerous tiny changes, some of which were favourable to the virus.

It's important to keep in mind that despite the 17 year gap between SARS and Covid-19, not that much changed in the virus code. Having examined the genetic code of the new virus and compared it with the original, the nomenclature committee chose to simply add the number 2. It was version 2 of the original.

This is what Nature tends to do. When a virus enters a new host species there might be a peak in mortalities, as seen with SARS. Nature then induces things to settle down. The new virus may never gain a true hold on the new species, and the two separate. Or the virus will adapt in such a way that it does not cause overt deaths and simply settles into a state of balance within the new host. Whether it kills each individual it infects depends on many factors. If something gives the virus an advantage it will certainly utilise that advantage.

By using alcohol hand sanitisers in the presence of Covid-19 patients, we will have ensured the solvent vapour rising from the sanitisers would enter the alveolar air sacks in which patients were replicating the virus. The target Alveolar Type 2 cells are covered by a special mucus called the pulmonary surfactant. It is this chemical mix that enables the air sacks to expand and contract on every breath.

Alcohol dissolves the chemical that makes up 40% of the pulmonary surfactant. That research was done on chemicals in a chemistry laboratory which some sceptics choose to say is not equivalent to human reality. So I choose to mention an old peer-reviewed article from the 1950s relating to an uncommon lung condition in which the pulmonary surfactant became a foam in the airways. People who developed this condition tended to die within hours of the foam forming as no oxygen could reach their blood. This was in the time when medicine was developing nebuliser drug delivery systems. They reported that when they nebulised 95% alcohol into the foam-blocked airways the alcohol broke down the foam and the patient lived (Reference 1). The alcohol broke down the pulmonary surfactant. The same pulmonary surfactant that protects our Alveolar Type 2 cells today. The very cells the Covid-19 coronavirus wants to attack.

The 1952 article means that we've had proof for well over half a century that alcohol dissolves pulmonary surfactant.

That means any alcohol vapour that reaches the alveolar air sacks has the capacity to weaken the mucus protection we expect to gain from the pulmonary surfactant. When the protection is diminished, the receptors on the target cells are easier to reach and the virus gains advantage. Each time the virus takes advantage and attacks an Alveolar Type 2 cell, more virus is replicated and more virus particles are released.

Unfortunately for infected people, it is the Alveolar Type 2 cells that make the pulmonary surfactant. Every such cell that is forced to make virus particles is one more cell that is no longer able to make pulmonary surfactant.

Every cell attacked means less protection for the cells around it. Every cell attacked means more virus particles to infect other cells or to be breathed out to infect other people.

All infections are dose dependent. Even vaccinated people can be infected if the number of infectious particles exceeds the level of protection generated by the vaccine. The key to preventing infections is to keep the number of infectious particles below the threshold required to infect the next person.

For much of this story we have discussed the virus taking advantage of the weakened pulmonary surfactant produced by the elderly. That is where I propose the SARS virus chose to go into balance. The fact that we did not see it over the intervening 16 years, during what I choose to call its shadow phase, means it was not infecting and killing younger people. It would have been infecting older people and if they died of bacterial pneumonia nobody would have had reason to suspect the involvement of an underlying virus.

That was the balance created by Nature under the laws of Nature. The new virus may have weakened the elderly to the point where the omnipresent bacterial pneumonia ended their lives. If so, that still fits the definition of balance in relation to the entire human population.

There was no natural reason for the adapted virus to suddenly kill hundreds of thousands of humans in a matter of months. That does not follow the laws of Nature. If that sudden change was not natural, we need to ask if humans were doing something unnatural which favoured the virus.

Solvent vapours emanating from alcohol hand sanitisers would allow for a strong thesis. This is a good time to stress that I am presenting a thesis. My dictionary defines thesis as: *"noun; a statement or theory that is put forward as a premise to be maintained or proved."* I would add that my thesis is put forward to be possibly disproved. My intention is to have it debated. If the debate goes against me I will return to the shadows and improve my thesis. If the debate goes for me I hope that hundreds of thousands of humans will be spared premature deaths.

The stakes are high. My dictionary defines stake in this context as: *"noun; a sum of money or something else of value gambled on the outcome of a risky game or venture."* I am gambling the valuable time it takes to write this book. National governments are gambling hundreds of thousands of lives. The stakes are indeed high. I can afford the time. Do the public want their government to gamble with their lives? I hope not, which is why I hope this book will generate sufficient public interest to become the momentum needed to move governments.

This book is a long way from being a PhD thesis in which I would expect to be examined by a panel of learned professors who needed to ensure I knew almost all there is to know about my chosen subject. I have a PhD and I know what such a panel-based oral examination entails. In my case it took place almost 40 years ago when I was called upon to defend my beliefs on what was happening in a new viral disease. I was granted my PhD by the Faculty of Medicine at the University of London. Since then I have dedicated my life to sharing ideas on how to prevent virus infections. I've been successful many times over many decades which provides the confidence to share new ideas on this virus here.

It was those new ideas I sought to share quietly with the UK Cabinet. The reason this book is being written is that I was unable to gain their attention in my favoured quiet fashion. Hopefully this book will draw the ideas to their attention so they can debate whether my ideas offer anything of value. While I am waiting for that to happen this book will spread the ideas among the public, and I must be content to hope someone passes the ideas to a member of the Cabinet and the debate begins.

The very high stakes make that a laudable ambition worthy of the time I'm gambling.

CHAPTER 9

At this mid-stage of the book, readers who are unaccustomed to what happens in the professional infection prevention world can be forgiven for hoping an obvious point like the solvent vapours would be addressed immediately. After all, we spend a lot of time telling children how unwise it is to sniff solvents, yet we are causing our Covid patients and their healthcare staff to do it in this time of heightened crisis.

Since there are ample hand sanitisers that have been proven effective yet do not liberate a solvent vapour, why not just switch to one of those?

I recall saying exactly that in the year 2000, although the subject related to the MRSA antibiotic-resistant superbug. I had worked closely with key influencers at a National Health Service (NHS) teaching hospital in the city where my company was located at the time. Together we had established how rarely healthcare workers performed hand hygiene and, in particular, how rarely the alcohol hand sanitiser was used. That meant the alcohol stayed in its bottle, never coming into contact with the superbug so the bug could go on infecting people.

Given that the collaboration included the hospital's infection control team and various healthcare workers, the alcohol-free product we were offering was actually something they had helped create.

Yet the hospital never took the product. When pushed to explain why, one of the main reasons given was that the WHO said to use alcohol. At that time the WHO was not actually saying that, but the stated reason was a viable excuse for doing nothing different. For many years that hospital continued to have a very sad infection rate.

In essence, patient outcome was not a high enough priority to require change. If that seems overly alarmist, consider that it was generally accepted that 5,000 patients would die each year in the UK from HealthCare Associated Infections (HCAI). Since it was accepted and expected, there was very little incentive to change.

I am firmly convinced that no one specific individual positively wanted the deaths to occur. It was more a collective consensus that since they were following what was deemed to be best practice they had done all that was required.

Before I go any further I would like to make it very clear that the hospital in question now, in 2020, has next to NO cases of MRSA infections. Their mindset changed, they took action and the patient outcomes improved. They showed it could be done with the correct mindset. This is not the place to explain what they changed. I simply want to ensure readers know they did.

However, for the first seven or eight years of this century I worked closely with them on several projects and they opted to utilise exactly none of the helpful findings. None of the other NHS hospitals in the UK that I was allowed to work with took any either.

It was becoming very clear that since they were not being inspired by what I considered to be appalling patient outcomes, it was best for them to just keep doing the same and expecting the same. They seemed perfectly content to appear too busy to prevent the deaths.

During that time I gave guest lectures at an international conference for the infection control profession. My forward-thinking positive perspective was always welcomed, and because I was always polite I received more invitations to speak. After all, there were always going to be thousands of deaths every year from hospital infections so it was worth talking about.

The one thing I could not induce them to discuss was the concept of making such infections rare events. I simply failed to move their mindsets to the point where that topic was even worth serious discussion.

Please accept this sequence as a recollection going back two decades. Some things have changed as demonstrated by the hospital results I have just presented. This sequence relates to what was happening and in many cases is still happening. Please do not judge all my hospital colleagues for their actions or lack thereof. It's best to appreciate that the professionals I was working with were doing the best they could with the resources they had available at the time. One of the resources they lacked was evidence that infections really could be made rare events. Since it had never happened in their working lives they had no reason to aim for that goal. They were very busy overcoming the inevitable infections they expected would occur, with no time left to contemplate how to stop the next infection happening.

From their perspective that was professionally justified. From their employer's perspective it was following evidence-based research and adhering to global gold standards.

From the patient perspective it was appalling.

I'm a very patient person yet even I decided it was time to move on. I had devoted a lot of professional thought and far too much commercial time attempting to advance the mindsets. It was just not happening.

Ironically my company was gaining half its revenue from the Republic of Korea where the mindset is fundamentally different.

My company began in my kitchen in 2001. As the kitchen reference implies, we began with little more than a professional understanding of how to prevent infections. I brought the base formulation from a previous company I had closed and we knew how to kill the problematic microbes.

One fundamental question underpinned our enthusiasm:

> "Since we know how to kill the microbes, why are the microbes still killing the people?"

The question was simple yet the connotations it triggered caused serious concern. We were fine with it because we were naive enough to assume that as soon as the appropriate cost-effective answer was presented it would be immediately incorporated into hospital policy. Unfortunately it was seen in the UK as being so simple that the hospital Boards would be castigated for not having done something similar years before. For a long time the NHS had the protection of Crown Immunity and could not be sued in courts. When that blanket immunity was removed the people paid to run hospitals had every justification for being afraid. They seemed to be more afraid of being sued for previous deaths than stepping out of line and preventing the next deaths.

They fell into a state of inertia very akin to the rabbit in the headlights we mentioned earlier. They could not go back and erase the needless deaths and, at the time, they could not see a way forward to prevent new ones. For far too many years they effectively did nothing and none of their employees felt inclined or safe to suggest otherwise.

I reluctantly took the decision to cease working so closely with the National Health Service. The new safe and effective products the hospital teams had helped us create were just too new and different. If they were used it could be seen to imply that the hospitals had been negligent in not using something similar before.

The problem was national mindset. In South Korea we met an entirely different mindset, and since 2008 half my company's revenue has been from exports to Korea. Financially I was secure thanks to the Koreans, yet I always remained ready to assist the UK National Health Service if a chance arose.

CHAPTER 10

The sudden Covid-19 event has given numerous companies an opportunity to rush in and make as much money as they can while we're in crisis. Fortunately there have also been some that sought to do good and help as much as they can. I've found myself being an advisor to the latter as they searched for individuals who had been influencing for a long time, people like myself who had a public record of always doing what was best even if it did take a long time. During 2020 I've spent a lot of good time repeating what you have just read in the previous chapter! If people entering the field for the first time were going to stand any chance of achieving their goals of making a positive contribution, it was important for them to know the facts and learn of any barriers to progress they were likely to encounter. It therefore behoves me to show that I am not a late entrant into the market seeking easy financial gain.

After being actively involved with the NHS for about a decade it became obvious my questions were becoming well known. It was equally obvious those same questions were beginning to annoy key influencers. Even though I was very well known as the person who really wanted to help patients achieve better outcomes, some key individuals in the health service did not like their bosses using my questions. It was time to step aside and approach from another direction.

When I opted to do so I realised how much really useful information had been shared with me by hard-working experienced healthcare workers. I had relied on their views for years, yet it was only when I collated it all that the true magnitude of it became apparent to me. Nurses, care staff and cleaners had been particularly forthcoming as it seemed I was the only person genuinely seeking their contributions. I was concerned that if I simply stepped aside to gain another approach angle I would be taking all that valuable information with me. It was obvious that if I began preaching about all the details, most people's eyes would glaze over within a few minutes.

I chose to weave it all into a novel on the presumption that if I made the novel exciting I would have the reader's attention for days.

In 2009 I published *The Reaper's Rainbow* to convey the few salient points a person entering hospital as a patient could use to ensure they did not become infected (Reference 2). I wrote it as an armageddon-type thriller with many people dying, as was happening in the hospitals. The story is set in the Board of an unidentified large UK teaching hospital; the sort I had been assisting at all levels for years and where I had seen working practices at the highest level. In the made-up story a new microbe begins killing patients and then advances to killing intensive-care nurses. The Chief Executive asks the hospital lawyer whether the deaths justify them changing their infection control procedures. The lawyer says no, they hadn't been sued the previous year for the infection deaths that occurred in their hospital so it would be very unwise to do anything different this time.

The reason I was relaxed about including such a callous concept in a novel is that I had heard it said while I was trying to help a major hospital end their infections. It represented a real-life event and epitomised the mindset that accompanies the actual deaths; the mindset I was still actively trying to shift. Nobody else was achieving that goal either so I knew it was nothing personal. There were simply too many obstacles to new ideas being acted upon. The recurring deaths from what I was suggesting were needless infections, simply did not warrant the hassle of change.

In the novel, I ramp up the pressure until the hospital Chief Executive finally decides to overrule his lawyer's advice. He decides that really new and draconian principles will be put in place; people are told to wash their hands and clean the floors. I had been trying to have them do that in real life for almost a decade with no success, so achieving it in a novel was a sneaky way of having it done.

On a lighter note, several months after publication I began to realise the sort of traps waiting for a first-time novelist. In the story, I took advantage of all the real deaths I'd learned of in real hospitals in order to allow numerous innocent members of the public to die for the sake of the story. It was fiction, yet in my view the only way I was going to force real-life change would be if I used the novelist's platform to kill enough people to make the horror noteworthy. As it happens I'm a positive person in real life and that had an effect on my storytelling in the novel. I chose to soften the horror slightly by including a budding relationship between two of the characters. After all, the story was one of great horror so surely little harm would arise from me taking off some of the sharp edges.

When people read it they began asking when I was doing a sequel to the love story. In their eyes the book belonged in the romance genre. That was a surprise to me as all the way through writing the novel I saw just an overriding disaster. Love has a wonderful way of shining through!

Sweet as that was to discover, one of the main themes in the 2009 novel was that alcohol hand sanitisers were not serving patients well. At the time there were many reasons why the hospitals around the world should have moved from alcohol to solvent-free sanitisers, and examples of those reasons will be seen in subsequent chapters. Yet none in the UK took that action. Some in South Korea have done so which allows me to prove our alternative product is both safe and effective. We've known that since 2009, yet alcohol sanitiser was still the favoured option when a new coronavirus arrived ten years later.

This time alcohol was more than an innocent bystander as it sat unused in its bottle. The terror surrounding Covid-19 was sufficient to have healthcare workers in Covid wards use a lot of alcohol, putting a lot of alcohol solvent vapour into the air and into the lungs of both Covid-19 victims and the workers themselves.

This time the solvent vapours from the alcohol sanitisers can arguably be called the culprit as the virus jumped from *natural* balance to *unnatural* pandemic.

I repeat for absolute clarity that my suggestion remains a thesis being presented for debate. However, one thing is certain. If the WHO had ceased suggesting the use of alcohol sanitisers when alternatives became available 20 years before, there would be no reason to present this thesis about alcohol vapours in 2020.

The WHO seems to have ignored the relevance of solvent vapours despite all the research publications on which cells these coronaviruses attack and other articles on how alcohol dissolves the pulmonary surfactant that should be protecting those lung cells.

That last sentence is deliberately simplistic and intentionally provocative. This book contains a lot of words including simplistic statements. Which of the latter touches the mind of the key influencer I am seeking is unknown, so I will use the statements to best effect.

It seems the WHO failed to tell us about the known relationship between solvent vapours and the pulmonary surfactant protecting the virus's target cells. In contrast it seems the coronavirus took full advantage of the obvious facts and found them very favourable.

If not the solvent vapours, what else helped the virus jump from balance to pandemic?

CHAPTER 11

I was very aware that publishing *The Reaper's Rainbow* was going to burn my metaphorical bridges with hospitals and the National Health Service. Why would anyone in that sector talk to me if I chose to share with the public the manner in which the system hid behind intransigent thinking with such callous disregard for the deaths of so many patients?

To my surprise and absolute delight, the novel rang true among several of my erstwhile infection prevention colleagues who were waiting for someone to step out and force a mindset change. These individuals agreed that the patient outcome statistics were appalling. However, being employees within the system made speaking out in such a manner very unwise.

On the basis of the novel I was invited to contribute a chapter in an infection prevention textbook. The invitation was a genuine validation of how my ideas were being appreciated in certain forward-thinking circles within the infection prevention profession. Far from burning my bridges, I was unwittingly creating new ones. The editor who commissioned my contribution gave me only one stipulation: that I should be provocative. He knew I would be polite, so provocative was safe.

INFECTION PREVENTION AND CONTROL: PERCEPTIONS AND PERSPECTIVES was published in 2016 (Reference 3). In the first paragraph of my chapter I wrote, "Change in something the HCAI profession has to use with due caution as change can bring new dangers. In this chapter, I will suggest failure to change presents greater danger than change."

The reality of how many infections were occurring every year was a feature of my contribution. It was impossible to say how many patients had been saved by what was generally called best practice. In sad and stark contrast, it was all too easy to say how many people had died from infection despite those best practices being in widespread use. There is a positive side. Even though the number of premature deaths from infections was appalling, when that number is seen in comparison with the overall number of patients, the best practices can be seen to have done a good job, statistically. It is, however, very unlikely a bereaved family would find much comfort in how many other patients had survived when their loved one died.

To them, best practice could be seen as best *failed* practice.

One of the biggest, and potentially unfairest, threats to infection control professionals is aggressive lawyers. The latter don't have to struggle under difficult conditions with limited resources achieving the near impossible every day. Lawyers have the tremendous advantage of hindsight as they tend to become involved after an unfortunate infection death has happened. Those lawyers can use the facts presented in the peer-reviewed medical articles to find gaps to attack.

When deaths from infections happen, healthcare professionals can be called upon to defend their hospital in court. One standard line of defence is to show they were following best practice and evidence-based research. That is fine if the lawyer will allow them to remain in the *technical* debate. However, the lawyer's aim is to convince lay members of the jury that it's more relevant to focus on the *outcome* debate. After all, the case is only being heard in court because of the poor outcome.

Should the lawyer who is defending the hospital decide to push the jury into the *technical* debate, things can be even worse for the hospital. People using the *technical* debate in their daily duties tend to point out how they are following evidence-based research. They are following the proven science. That of course is intended to be a convincing argument and it carries weight during discussions in hospitals. It can be disastrous in court.

While preparing to write the chapter, I allocated myself three hours to read articles in one well-known British infection control journal. I chose to read it from the perspective of an aggressive lawyer; someone who wanted to have the jury question the validity of the *technical* debate. If you want details of what I found please read the actual chapter. For now, suffice it to say that it was very easy to find peer-reviewed, evidence-based research that proved just how bad things were. It would be very easy for an aggressive lawyer to ask the jurors whether the hospital team had been following evidence of success or evidence of *failure*? The medical articles I cite in the chapter provided evidence of failure.

The patient in this hypothetical court case can be shown to have died as a result of persistent failures inherent within the supposed best practice. Or at least it's safe to say any good lawyer who had bothered to read the relevant medical literature would find it easy to bring a jury to that conviction.

At this vital juncture please keep in mind that I am a positive person and my chapter in the textbook serves a positive purpose. That is why I was invited to contribute. In the chapter, I invite infection control professionals to combine the three main topics of debate: namely *technical, outcome and financial*. All three are common subjects, yet they are usually seen as separate entities. Infection control professionals spend a lot of time augmenting the technical aspects while lamenting how often they see unfavourable outcomes.

In the *technical* debate the focus is on microbes dying; in the *outcome* debate it's on people dying. That distinction can be devastating to the morals of caring professionals who are doing all they can every day.

All of this, they often suggest, could be helped by more resources, especially more human resources. To them that lies in the *financial* debate. Very few infection control professionals spend much of their scarce spare time thinking they might be able to influence the financial debate, as they believe it only takes place in the main hospital Boardroom.

Yet the largest human resource in most hospitals is the patients. They:

- tend to be of an age that provides them with broad and diverse experiences of life
- have a lot of spare time
- agree that infections in patients are less than favourable, and best of all
- don't need to be paid.

This patient cohort, this massive untapped human resource, can be utilised without the Board members being involved. It would help if the latter wanted to be involved, yet their participation is far from necessary.

My mention here of the chapter from this infection control textbook is intended to serve three purposes:

1. To show the forward-thinking ideas I generate are valued by the forward thinkers.
2. To explain why the principles of infection prevention currently used fail to serve us well.
3. To emphasise to you, the reader, that things need to change and that change is most likely to arise when the public rise up against the appalling outcomes.

Hospitals in the UK are fundamentally under the control of the government. If favourable changes are to happen, they are likely to only occur when the public induce the government to change.

Fortunately there is a very simple way to overcome the whole healthcare associated infection problem. As you might imagine after reading this far into the book, alcohol hand sanitisers are absent in the new principles, and solvent vapours do not arise from any of the products used. I will share that elsewhere as it's too far removed from the main subject of this particular book.

For now suffice it to say that the number of Covid-19 victims who died from coronavirus infections caught at work warrants our complete attention.

CHAPTER 12

If alcohol hand sanitisers can be shown to represent such failed technology over many years in hospitals, why were they suggested as a vital tool to combat the coronavirus which came to our attention in Wuhan? That is and will remain a key question.

The medical evidence so often quoted as a means of support by the authorities and influencers, actually contains a huge amount of evidence on how alcohol *failed* to stop even simple bacterial infections. What they are perpetuating as evidence of success is actually evidence of failure. Alcohol hand sanitisers were introduced in the 1950s. That means infection control professionals employed anywhere in the world today are placing great reliance on something that the medical evidence reveals has been failing patients since before those employees were first employed. It is fair to say alcohol in this context is a failed technology. It is grossly unfair to say the people are career failures. It's unfair because most of them had little option. They were told to use alcohol sanitisers and this year they were so scared of Covid-19 they chose to do as they were told.

Blame is a very expensive verb. Returning to my trusted dictionary, I find the following definition of blame: *"verb; feel or declare that (someone or something) is responsible for a fault or wrong."* Thousands of deaths every year from needless bacterial infections over many decades most definitely constitutes a fault or wrong. Hundreds of thousands of Covid-19 deaths in less than a year is even worse.

Which induces me to repeat the statement that blame is a very expensive verb. Obviously the word itself is not at fault. The problem and subsequent costs arise when we use the word. When we opt to blame someone or something we can become the fault or wrong.

The original SARS virus killed many thousands of people, so blame can be apportioned; especially since people like me can now trawl through the evidence. Yet what do we gain by introducing blame? Do we benefit by blaming:

- bats which still host the virus
- civet cats for apparently passing the virus to humans
- the people running the wet markets in China where the virus was supposed to have jumped species into humans?

In my view we do not benefit from blame. Our gain comes when we benefit from learning what happened and using that new knowledge to prevent such things happening again. When the Covid-19 coronavirus broke out, many chose to blame the Chinese wet markets again. That was an easy thing to do and anyone who felt inclined to favour blame in that manner has had ample time to wonder how well they were served by that blame game.

Should the debate on my thesis go in my favour, the use of alcohol hand sanitisers as part of infection prevention best practice will be shown to be instrumental in bringing us the current pandemic.

The whole Covid-19 sequence is so monumental I prefer to avoid blame which might become focused by others into areas we subsequently find less useful.

However, we do owe an obligation to all those who have been adversely affected by Covid-19 to examine the evidence we chose to trust and follow. If we have genuinely been following evidence of failure there is a cultural matter to consider.

Over many weeks, members of the UK Cabinet were seen in their daily television Covid-19 news briefings. They did their best to keep us all informed in a rapidly changing calamity. They were telling us they were following the science provided by their scientific and medical advisors. They were correctly watching what was happening in other nations and using that evidence to chart what they saw as the best course for the UK. Put very simply, these beleaguered politicians were doing the best they could with the resources they had available at the time. Yet they had to stand there in full public view sharing some frighteningly horrific and sad statistics of so many individual lives lost.

Which makes it appropriate to examine some of the evidence they had available. I will deliberately select one example that shows what they were up against, one piece of evidence I found of particular interest.

On 12 April 2020 their Global Death Comparison chart mentioned eight countries. On that day the UK trajectory was exactly on the line for Italy. It was known that the UK was two weeks behind Italy and yet we were choosing to do the same as Italy was doing. We were being guided by the science Italy had experienced. On that date, almost 20,000 Italians were recognised to have died from Covid-19, whereas China had lost about 3,000. That comparison suggests failure on Italy's part, and the UK chose to follow Italy and do what was being done in Italy rather than take the lead from China.

I present this analysis and opinion based on that one day's statistics to demonstrate what the Cabinet members were having to deal with on a daily basis. What would other politicians have done if asked to decide on that day with the same resources? Probably something similar.

History can choose to judge the UK Cabinet more harshly if it wants. I prefer to ask how I can help the members of that same Cabinet with the many choices they still have to face for the remainder of 2020 and into 2021.

The main choice I want them to consider is removing alcohol hand sanitisers for at least the duration of the Covid-19 pandemic. In my view there is simply too much proven medical and scientific evidence to suggest solvent vapours from alcohol sanitisers could be favouring the Covid-19 coronavirus.

CHAPTER 13

The fact that I am presenting so much to dissuade people from advocating the use of alcohol sanitisers makes it worth mentioning a few of the many medical facts that have long supported that view. There has been concern over alcohol for many decades, with my thesis of its involvement in the pathogenesis of Covid-19 simply being a new component.

Alcohol sanitisers make use of the excellent antimicrobial effect of liquid alcohol. To achieve the appropriate level of antimicrobial effectiveness sanitisers must contain a minimum proportion of alcohol, usually designated as 70% alcohol in water. Gelling agents are usually added to ensure the product stays on the hands rather than running off them.

The liquid alcohol is known to have evaporated from the hands in about 15 seconds. Therefore the liquid alcohol has that brief time in which to act against microbes. There are too many authoritative published articles on the kill rate of 70% alcohol to present them here. A simple way to summarise them is to present the technical aspects of the European protocol for antimicrobial hand sanitisers. EN1500 is the test to determine how the efficacy of a new alcohol sanitiser compares to that of 70% ethanol. In the test procedure, hands are first cleaned and then contaminated with a very large number of bacteria. To pass EN1500, the alcohol-based test product is required to remove 100,000 bacteria before the liquid alcohol from a single application has evaporated.

The combination of the very high number of microbes to be killed and the short duration in which the liquid alcohol remains on the hands are the pertinent aspects that make alcohol worthy of debate.

At this stage it is very important to stress that alcohol sanitisers that pass the EN1500 test are extremely effective at killing certain microbes on the hands. This book relates to the Covid-19 coronavirus, and alcohol sanitisers are extremely efficient at killing that virus. If the only requirement was to kill that pathogen, it would have been correct to advocate the use of alcohol sanitisers to deliver protection during this pandemic.

However, this chapter relates to the effectiveness of alcohol sanitisers in general. I have been suggesting all alcohol sanitisers should have been replaced with other products that contain active ingredients which remain on the hands. For those products only the water they contain evaporates.

The key reasons being that certain common pathogens are not killed by alcohol in the very brief few seconds the liquid alcohol is on the skin. The most common of these pathogens is Norovirus which causes very common outbreaks of vomiting and diarrhoea in hospitals, schools, care homes and cruise ships. A solution of 70% alcohol will kill Norovirus if contaminated hands are immersed in the alcohol for long enough. However, when alcohol is applied to hands the active ingredient evaporates before it has time to complete the killing process. Since only an extremely small number of virus particles are required for Norovirus to infect a person, the fact that viable virus particles are expected to be left on hands becomes a very significant issue.

For many decades after Norovirus became an issue, NHS hospitals continued to advocate the use of alcohol sanitisers during outbreaks of Noroviral disease. One particular London hospital stood apart by removing alcohol sanitisers during outbreaks and making available a small leaflet explaining the reason to patients.

This is relevant here to demonstrate how the infection prevention profession and its employers can continue with a practice they know does not prevent infection. I believed this blatant disregard needed to be brought to the attention of the public. The fact that I was doing so drew my attention to the fact that my questions were causing annoyance among the professionals I was trying to help. To openly ask people to apply a flammable solvent to their hands during a Norovirus outbreak in hospitals when it was known to be ineffective was, in my view, a blatant act of deception. That was my view then and it remains my view now.

Fortunately this deceptive practice ceased several years ago and now the whole medical sector advocates the use of hand washing at a basin during Norovirus outbreaks rather than extra use of alcohol sanitisers. Yet few hospitals have provided extra hand washing stations or provided their busy staff with extra time to conduct the hand washing procedure. One step forward in the medical sector acknowledging, and moving on from, a long-heralded falsehood. Two steps backwards as the busy staff could not perform appropriate hygiene.

The salutary lesson is how long the medical profession was prepared to advocate the use of a hazardous product when in at least one major hospital everyone was being told very publicly it did not work.

Alcohol hand sanitisers are still used on cruise ships during Norovirus outbreaks. For a number of years I was instrumental in reducing the impact of Norovirus on the ships in several small cruise lines. That was done by first removing the alcohol sanitisers and replacing them with another hand sanitiser that left the active ingredient on treated hands. The other actions taken relate to floors and surfaces and are best discussed elsewhere. The pertinent point is that the small cruise lines believed the Norovirus outbreaks were adversely affecting their commercial reputations so they took specific actions to replace alcohol sanitisers. The larger cruise lines seemed to have a view that such outbreaks were expected by their passengers so they simply sailed on. The fact the companies knew alcohol sanitisers do not kill Norovirus in their setting seems to be deemed irrelevant. Their paying guests expect Norovirus outbreaks to occur on cruise ships and those same passengers expect to have ample alcohol sanitisers provided when an outbreak occurs. Under the axiom that it pays to meet expectations, it makes good commercial sense for the cruise lines to continue providing an ineffective product and disregard the obvious physical discomfort of passengers who develop vomiting and diarrhoea while on a cruise.

We still sell our alcohol-free hand sanitiser to cruise companies for use by passengers who say they cannot tolerate alcohol sanitisers. The cruise companies have assessed our product and acknowledge it meets their requirements in combatting Norovirus. It just fails to satisfy their desire to meet customer expectations.

Alcohol also evaporates from hands before it has killed bacterial spores. This became especially relevant with the rise of *Clostridium difficile* outbreaks in wards containing elderly patients. The condition caused by this bacterium effectively rots the bowels of infected patients leading to a lethal diarrhoea with a particularly characteristic stench. There is no nice way to describe it. For decades alcohol sanitisers were advocated for use during *Clostridium difficile* outbreaks even though it was known the active alcohol evaporated from hands before it had killed all the spores.

Fortunately the thinking has moved on and now extra hand washing is advocated. This is yet another example of bad practice being part of what the hospital system used to assure the public was best practice.

CHAPTER 14

Employers must protect workers and others from getting hurt or ill through work. In the UK the rules are outlined in the Health and Safety Executive (HSE) page https://www.hse.gov.uk/riddor/occupational-diseases.htm.

Employers are required to inform the HSE of any occupational disease, of which occupational dermatitis is a prevalent example. If an employer fails to report, a regulator such as the HSE or local authority may take action under criminal law. There is absolutely no doubt under the law that occupational dermatitis should be taken seriously.

Which raises the question of whether it actually is taken seriously enough. There is a plethora of published medical articles going to great lengths over decades to say the hand hygiene products commonly used in UK hospitals are safe and do not cause occupational dermatitis. The work is extensive, is often repetitive and costs a huge amount of money. Why would the healthcare sector allocate such amounts when they are chronically short of financial resources? Why are they publishing so many articles if there is not a fundamental issue?

Why indeed. Having watched the growth of this publishing bonanza over two decades I'm reminded of the many papers published by the tobacco industry when they were trying to claim there were no health hazards from smoking tobacco. More recently the food industry has been publishing numerous articles implying they have no role in the obesity epidemic. Both of those industry sectors have large profits to pour into numerous publications.

The healthcare sector, and in particular the NHS, frequently says it needs more cash to achieve the desired level of patient care. That demonstrates why it is so relevant for the public to know why so much money is being allocated to all these studies. For decades the articles have suggested alcohol hand sanitisers are not the primary cause of the occupational dermatitis so prevalent among healthcare workers. Whether that is a smoke-screen denial akin to those used by the tobacco and food industries can be discussed elsewhere.

For now let's take them at their word and for a moment ignore how much valuable money has been spent in arriving at that decision. We are still left with the fact that, for generations, hospital hand hygiene, of which alcohol hand sanitisers are a very significant part, has allowed hundreds of thousands of patients to die premature deaths through infections. Alcohol hand sanitisers play a part in that failed technology.

Last century that statement might have left the NHS without suitable hand hygiene products. Since the year 2000, perfectly effective alcohol-free alternative products have been available. Our versions are constantly used in NHS hospitals, although only for staff who have obvious occupational dermatitis and therefore can't use the traditional products. That raises more questions. If those traditional products, including alcohol sanitisers, were not the cause of the occupational dermatitis, why switch those sufferers to our products? Perhaps even more important, if our products have been deemed effective enough for use by people with dermatitis, then those products are suitable for use throughout the hospital. There are now brands in addition to ours which do not contain alcohol, so this paragraph should be taken as generic. I can speak about our products because I invented them and we have 20 years of excellent results. Other suppliers will speak for their own products.

The point is that the healthcare sector has absolutely no technical reason to continue using failed technology which has allowed the loss of so many lives.

In recent years the microbiome of an individual has become topical. Microbiologists have been using the term for a long time and it has finally found a public space. Part of the overall microbiome is the biome of the skin on hands. It is generally accepted that it pays to leave the biome to take care of itself which implies the avoidance of antimicrobial products with the capacity to kill more microbes than is required.

Many purchasing decisions on hand sanitisers in the UK are based on whether the product passes the EN1500 test. Any product that does is capable of killing 100,000 bacteria on hands on one application. We have already discussed that alcohol sanitisers can achieve that, and now there are some alcohol-free products that achieve the same. If all you were seeking to do is meet marketing expectations, that might appear as a useful contribution.

However, that would avoid clinical facts. If there is visible soiling on hands, the person is expected to use a hand wash at a basin. They should not be using a hand rub, commonly called hand sanitiser, which is left on the hands to dry. In the absence of visible soil, the person is left to assume the hand rub will achieve the antimicrobial objective. EN1500 compliant products will certainly be capable of removing 100,000 bacteria.

Sadly, or perhaps happily, there are usually only 100 bacteria on clinically clean hands. This is demonstrated by the requirement in the USA for a hand rub, a hand sanitiser, to prove it can remove 100 bacteria in one use and 1,000 in ten successive uses. The Americans have used the clinical setting as their guide, whereas in the UK the EN1500 test has erroneously become dominant. That means any product that can pass EN1500 is coming with the capacity for a thousand times overkill. Obviously they can't kill the same bacterium 1,000 times which leaves that massive spare capacity to act against the helpful microbiome on the user's hands as well. Whether that translates into problems for the user will be determined in time.

The point is that hand hygiene products that have the capacity to address the clinical microbial load exist, which means neither flammable solvents nor 1,000 times overkill from alcohol-free products need be tolerated.

CHAPTER 15

COSHH is the law that requires UK employers to control substances that are hazardous to health.

If the packaging has any of the hazard symbols then the product is classed as a hazardous substance, as suggested on the HSE site https://www.hse.gov.uk/coshh/basics/substance.htm.

Alcohol sanitisers must, by law, have hazard symbols on the packaging, proving beyond doubt that they are classed as hazardous. Those hazard symbols mean it is the liquid alcohol within the container which is hazardous. Whether that translates into clinical disease in the form of occupational dermatitis has been discussed adequately in a previous chapter. On balance, given the weight of articles in which so many authors strove to reach the same conclusion, the liquid alcohol is not the primary cause of occupational dermatitis on the hands of healthcare workers.

The one point which is set in law is that the hazard symbols on the containers confirm alcohol sanitisers to be hazardous under COSHH. That alone is reason to at least examine the obligation under COSHH to consider substituting it. The thesis that this hazard triggered and then possibly fuelled the current pandemic adds to that obligation.

The following sentence and the list of seven steps are taken from the same HSE website:

"You can prevent exposure to a hazardous substance by substituting it with another substance which presents less, or no risk.

There are seven steps to practical, well thought out decisions about substitution.

1. Decide whether the substance or process is a hazard. Is there a significant risk involved in storing, using or disposing of a substance?
2. Identify the alternatives.
3. Think about what could happen if you use the alternatives.
4. Compare the alternatives with each other and with the substance or process you are using at the moment.
5. Decide whether to substitute.
6. Introduce the substitute.
7. Assess how it is working."

Substitutes for alcohol hand sanitisers exist and are already in use around the world. They are effective and safe. In this context substitution of hazardous alcohol sanitisers can happen now.

The mere fact that a substance is classed as hazardous does not mean it must be substituted. As is stated in the same website: "If you can't prevent exposure, you need to control it adequately by applying the principals of good control practice. Control is adequate when the risk of harm is 'as low as is reasonably practicable.'"

Since alcohol as a hand sanitiser can so easily be argued to be failed technology from the patient outcome perspective, and substituting it is already done in many hospitals, it seems a poor use of resources to go through the processes of good control practices required by COSHH if you decide to continue using that hazardous substance.

The solvent vapour rising from hands to which the liquid alcohol has been applied is another matter. There are many medical articles, two of which are mentioned in subsequent paragraphs, which prove the vapour is breathed in and passes through the alveolar wall into the blood. That solvent vapour is not packaged and cannot carry hazard icons. However, since it is a direct consequence of alcohol sanitiser being used, the latter is deemed to have delivered the hazardous vapour. The weight of argument in the many articles is that the solvent alcohol vapour breathed in is also not associated with conditions that might be considered dangerous.

The new point which arose in 2020 is the possibility that, over an extended period of many years, one specific virus progressively adapted to the advantage provided by solvent alcohol vapours as the ethanol decreased the effectiveness of pulmonary surfactant protection on the alveolar walls. This concept is conjecture, as must be repeated yet again. If the debate over my thesis goes in my favour, the horrendous effect of the Covid-19 pandemic will be deemed to have been triggered in a large part by the effect of solvent alcohol vapour which arose from hands treated with alcohol sanitisers. The mere mention of that sequence is sufficient to warrant examining the hazardous nature of alcohol hand sanitisers.

Therefore the vapour from alcohol hand sanitisers must be considered from the COSSH perspective. By now you might agree with me that, at the very least, this is becoming a potential waste of resources when there are so many reasons to simply substitute the hazardous substance to which the hazard symbols refer. If you are still wondering whether change is warranted, consider the following wording from a COSHH safety data sheet for ethanol from a very reputable supplier. Under the section for respiratory protection is the statement: "Follow the OSHA respirator regulations found in 29 CFR 1910.134 or European Standard EN 149. Use a NIOSH/MSHA or European Standard EN 149 approved respirator if exposure limits are exceeded or if irritation or other symptoms are experienced."

You could spend valuable resources following the detailed steps set out in those last two sentences, or you could substitute the alcohol sanitiser with a product known around the world to be effective and safe.

There are many medical articles relating to alcohol vapour arising from alcohol hand sanitisers used on hands being breathed in by the user. One in the *Journal of Hospital Infection* revealed how alcohol breathed out within one to two minutes of using an alcohol hand sanitiser was detectable using a breathalyser (Reference 4). The alcohol could not be detected 15 minutes after use of the sanitiser so the product was deemed to be safe from the legal perspective. However, this article graphically demonstrates that alcohol vapour rising from hand sanitisers is definitely breathed in by the user.

Another article, in the *Forensic Science International* journal (Reference 5), proved ethanol from hand sanitisers is incorporated by the respiratory tract but not via the skin. They detected a specific chemical marker for alcohol in the urine, which proved the alcohol had come from the hand sanitiser, via the lungs, into the blood, been metabolised, and this chemical marker was then detectable in the urine as it was being excreted from the body. The key point is that alcohol from the alcohol hand sanitisers had crossed the alveolar wall, which means it *had* gone through the pulmonary surfactant layer.

Many other articles relate to the fact that ethanol that is drunk passes out from the blood via the alveolar wall to the alveolar air space. Alcohol molecules passing in that direction decrease the protective effect of the pulmonary surfactant (Reference 6). That places even greater pressure on employers' obligations to substitute alcohol sanitisers if the employers know or reasonably suspect their employees who work in a clinical Covid setting are likely to consume alcoholic drinks. This will form a significant part of the debate I want my thesis to generate as this additional alcohol is known to reduce the effectiveness of pulmonary surfactant and the lung's ability to remove infectious debris (Reference 7).

It is still the same ethanol molecule regardless of whether it is passing from the alveolar space into the blood or in the reverse direction. In both cases it passes through the pulmonary surfactant that innately defends ACE2 receptors on Alveolar Type 2 cells from attack by SARS-CoV-2.

In itself, my thesis that solvent vapours arising from the use of alcohol sanitisers favour replication of the virus deep within lungs, does not place an immediate legal obligation on employers to substitute the hazardous product. My hope is that the debate arising from challenging my thesis will bring forth data and momentum to make it an obligation.

The debate must happen first and in order to trigger that debate my thesis must be presented in such a way that the debate occurs. The major obligation is on me at the moment to induce the debate and thereby lead to alcohol sanitisers being substituted.

CHAPTER 16

I have gone to some length in showing numerous reasons why alcohol sanitisers could be deemed to be failed technology and should be substituted for the sake of patient safety. That could have been done before SARS ever existed and the time between SARS and Covid-19 simply reinforces the pressure.

I spend most of my time working with non-medical people and I'm often asked why the doctors don't simply take the easier option and get on with substituting alcohol sanitisers. One of the simplest ways to shut down my debate would be to do the substitution. It has already been done in a small number of hospitals around the world over the last 20 years without negative effect. Then why is the hazardous substance still in use at all? Why would the WHO advocate alcohol's widespread use when there are so many reasons to substitute it?

Reluctance to change is one major reason. The medical profession is well known to take its time in implementing change. It is far from being alone among professions in this regard, although that is far from being a valid reason for such intransigence. Busy professionals who must be completely focused on their speciality by the nature of their work, often lack the skills or reason to consider wider aspects. This is a prominent factor in many professions and is represented very well in the concept of Diseases of Meaning (Reference 8). Disease and health are often thought of as distinct opposites, yet when a broader perspective is taken it can be seen how they relate to each other. This is a relatively new realisation in what is generally called Western medicine. If the thesis presented in this book survives the intended debate, it will be seen how Covid deaths follow a sequence whereby infection occurred, a previously unrecognised danger to patients in the form of solvent vapours became involved, and the patients died. The "disease", which we see as deaths, becomes the end point of a sequence that includes the decision to ignore the solvent vapour rising from the hand sanitisers. The action that will prevent the disease, the deaths, involves substituting the alcohol sanitisers. In this context, the decision to use such products was a fundamental component of the disease pathogenesis, and the patients were unwittingly turned into victims of that decision.

UK law provides an obligation to consider substituting hazardous alcohol sanitisers, and the many clinical reasons I've listed in this text suggest the best defence would be to substitute such products. This book would not exist if the hazardous substance which liberates solvent vapours into the lungs of users and patients had been substituted as soon as viable substitutes were available. That could have happened pre-SARS and, if it had been done, I ask would Covid-19 have existed? Who can say, yet the question certainly generates intrigue.

A non-medical reader can be forgiven for wondering why they won't just get on with it. In response to that I would like to offer a glimmer of support for the medical profession.

To put it frankly, they function in a very complex arena. Change in one aspect can create problems in another and since there are so many inter-connected facets it can be incredibly difficult. In contrast, change in other sectors and industries can be easier to implement as there are far fewer interlocking matters. If I want to make changes in my factory, there are usually just a few other matters to consider. If the medical profession wants to substitute alcohol sanitisers there are a vast number of other factors to consider.

That's why I'm only prepared to offer a *glimmer* of support. Yes, it's complex and they knew that when they accepted the job. Failure to consider all the consequences can be revealed in the number of patient deaths. The stakes are high. Families bereaved by an infection death should not be expected to find good in the system that might have played a part in allowing their loved one to die. If people want to be paid to do this job, they take it upon themselves to do it safely.

That is deliberately abrupt. It's a matter of tough medicine, and as patients we often need to accept tough medicine. The doctors prescribe it in the belief it is good for us. I prescribe it to them here in the same belief. When something useful is just beyond their appreciation it's mutually beneficial to have it pointed out as an available choice. Being told to do something rarely works to mutual benefit. However, being shown something useful while being encouraged to see it as a viable choice delivers far better outcomes. Should the recipient choose to ignore the other choice, *de facto* they take it upon themselves to justify any negative consequences like patients dying premature deaths.

Again I would like to help by demonstrating how this can be a genuine matter of perspective. If you lined ten infection control professionals up in front of a hospital with the usual number of infection deaths, they will probably give you ten valid science-based reasons for the patient outcomes. If you lined ten members of the public up and asked them, you would probably hear ten things that could be changed. All 20 would favour fewer infections, yet the first ten are constrained by limiting beliefs gained via learned experiences.

I would now like to present an example of how the mindset widely encountered in medicine can be the barrier to change. Thinking without sufficient regard to other aspects can become the source of a problem. This example is being presented mainly to show non-medical people how long it can take to correct what could be interpreted as an apparent error.

In 2009, the Royal College of Physicians published an extensive paper titled *Dermatitis: Occupational aspects of management: Evidence-based guidance for healthcare professionals* (Reference 9). When I was doing my research for this book I went in search of a more recent version and was intrigued to see the shortened version available for download. What was being advocated in 2009 was still being advocated in 2020.

I wish to begin by saying the document's contents are thorough and a very good contribution to the advancement of medicine. It was the first time I had seen an official acceptance that hand hygiene products, and particularly hand washes, were the cause of so much occupational dermatitis. Prior to that, anyone who suggested such a thing was usually met with aggressive challenges and denial. The 2009 document meant those of us who were accustomed to being challenged in that fashion had official support for our long-held ideas. In essence it is a useful, constructive document. So why am I citing it here?

The answer lies in recommendation 8 of the shortened version. It says: "If a patient who works in healthcare has hand dermatitis that is caused or made worse by work, you should advise them to use alcohol rubs ...." In itself that statement shows due regard for the fact that when dermatitis is caused by hand washes it is reasonable to allow the sufferer to avoid using hand washes. It also takes due regard of the healthcare setting and the need to ensure workers take all actions to avoid inadvertently transferring microbes to those they are caring for at the time. So it looks fine from those perspectives.

Now I ask you to consider what happens when someone puts a flammable solvent onto damaged skin? *It causes harm.* As was stressed in the previous chapter, alcohol sanitisers are hazardous substances. By telling employees with dermatitis to apply alcohol rub to their damaged skin, the employer is *telling the employees to harm themselves* with a substance known by the employer to be hazardous. I will avoid going into details on the many very serious legal consequences of that action.

That is a good example of where complications can so easily arise in the complex field of medicine. I still favour this 2009 document as it takes us a long way forward. However, a blatant mismatch appeared in the recommendations. The recommendation that employers should effectively advise their employees to damage themselves is very wrong.

One of the suggestions they could have made in 2009 was that the employees be advised to use a hand rub that did not contain a flammable solvent. Such products were well known at the time and they had been in regular use in some UK hospitals by staff with hand dermatitis. Unfortunately the original document said alcohol rub should be advised.

Please accept this chapter in its intended guise as me attempting to enable the system to come to its own realisation that it has other choices and arguably an obligation to take them. My intention here is to reveal choices.

I hope non-medical readers will appreciate it as an example of how good progress in one area of medicine can result in problems elsewhere. Such unforeseen negative outcomes can impede positive attempts to consider and instigate change. It can reinforce an aversion to change. Had that 2009 paper suggested ALL healthcare workers use alcohol-free rubs regardless of dermatitis, this book would not be needed. In my thesis I imply the current pandemic may even not have occurred if alcohol vapours were not virtually ubiquitous in the Covid-19 clinical setting.

That is a bold statement. I ask readers to consider what else might have advanced the virus from a state of co-existence and balance into a pandemic if not solvent alcohol vapours? If you know of, or can legitimately propose, something else that could have achieved that, please let me know.

CHAPTER 17

We are now entering the final part of the book. So let's ask what could happen if the issues we've discussed are ignored?

Perhaps this is the best time to present the many reasons why I feel the UK is heading for a true catastrophe in the coming winter if we continue as we are. All of the points in the following sequence are deliberate over-simplifications, as I am doing my best to present a dystopian view. I hope to shock the system into hearing of, and adopting, a choice that it is currently failing both to see and utilise. New factors may well arise which are not apparent to me as I write this in August 2020. Unfortunately what you will see presented in this chapter is ample to generate the desired dystopian view.

I will begin with school children and in particular primary school children in the first years of school. We know comparatively little of their role in spreading this coronavirus although we do know they shed it (Reference 10). Even if only a low proportion of them become spreaders, the sheer number of them makes the impact of their potential combined spreading effect a significant threat to society.

When UK children go back to school after their summer break, they will cease to be restricted within their family groups. Multiple family groups will be mixed in each classroom, favouring cross contamination with the coronavirus. As a society we have finally achieved excellent hand hygiene manners in young children, especially children in primary school. When the current cohort of primary school children return to school they will use alcohol sanitisers diligently and inadvertently breathe in solvent vapours rising from those products. Very few, if any, of those children will develop the respiratory symptoms of Covid-19. However, we know some will become infected and shed the virus. I argue that the more alcohol vapour they breathe in, the more virus each infected child is likely to produce and breathe out.

Those young children will shed the virus in their homes. Parents know how common it is for them to become infected by viruses their children bring home from school. That has been happening for a very long time. The only change in 2020 is that the pandemic coronavirus could be among the viruses transferred from children to their parents. The statistical chance of any of these parents developing Covid-19 symptoms is quite low, which partly explains why they are showing an increasing reluctance to remain constrained by the Covid safety guidelines. This group also tends to be enthusiastic users of alcohol sanitisers, partly as the means of reinforcing good hygiene practices in their young children. Should the parents become infected, their use of alcohol sanitisers could increase the amount of virus their infected lung cells produce, meaning more virus is breathed out by the parents. Since it's unlikely they will have clinical symptoms, any tendencies they have for paying less regard to Covid precautionary guidelines will exacerbate the number of people they can infect outside their homes.

Fortunately for the pupils, teachers will go about their duties in a professional manner. Unfortunately for the teachers, they will find it very hard to avoid any virus being shed by their pupils. Preventive measures like social distancing will be adhered to as well as they can be with young children. However, I have yet to hear any reference as to whether the required distance between people includes consideration of wind direction. Being one metre upwind of a person who is shedding coronavirus could be a lot safer than being two metres downwind of the same person. This is a very simple fact which is rarely discussed.

Teachers use a lot of alcohol sanitisers while protecting themselves and continuing their valiant efforts to instil good hygiene practices in their pupils. The age of teachers can extend well into the range where Covid-19 symptoms are more common. There is great diversity among teachers and they will include individuals with comorbidities known to be associated with an increased chance of being infected by the virus, shedding the virus and becoming ill with Covid-19. Teachers are taking personal risks in performing their role among pupils who will undoubtedly be shedding the Covid coronavirus.

It is therefore a reasonable expectation that some teachers will die from Covid-19 if the current situation prevails throughout winter.

There is now a lot more of the Covid coronavirus circulating in the UK than there was before the lockdown in spring. Then we needed people to bring the virus into the country, whereas now we have many thousands of people multiplying the virus here and spreading it in their respective communities. Having that much more virus increases the chance of multiplying the number of virus particles, breathing out more virus, and any individual becoming infected.

Face coverings are reminding most people there is an issue to be considered. However, it is well known that most face coverings do not stop the majority of virus particles being breathed out nor the majority of virus particles being breathed in. As time progresses, enforcing adherence to face-covering instructions could become a challenge in our culture.

It has been reported that the end of lockdown is being interpreted by many people as the end of the problem. The Government has a huge communication challenge to ensure people remain as aware as they need to be. Prior to the lockdown, advisors to the Government were stressing that instructions for social compliance would have reduced effectiveness over time. That is proving to be true. Enough people convincing themselves and their contacts that the problem has gone away will increase the chance of an even greater calamity in the very near future.

Even though several million UK residents have been infected with the coronavirus, over 90% of the population remains fully susceptible to infection. We may be in for some good news when antibody tests become more widespread. However, until then we need to appreciate that most people are yet to be infected. A report published in mid-August 2020 suggested that 6% of the UK population had been infected by the coronavirus. To people like me who work to prevent virus problems, 6% is far too close to zero. In epidemiological terms we might as well assume the population is just as susceptible as it was at the beginning of the year. We are a very long way from the much heralded herd immunity, which means that in practical terms we are just as susceptible as a population now as we were at the beginning, and at a time when there is a lot more virus.

The Government is claiming to be dismissing the option of a national lockdown in the case of a significant resurgence of coronavirus infections and Covid-19 deaths. They have opted for local restrictions with local lockdowns when necessary. Given the amount of confusion that arose during the one national lockdown, multiple local lockdowns may induce even more confusion. Time will tell whether that confusion favours the pandemic here in the UK resulting in many more deaths.

Furloughed workers had a financial incentive to remain in strict lockdown. The ending of that scheme is likely to coincide with many employers going out of business. Prior to Covid many companies lacked sufficient cash to pay for loans. Companies who were in that state then, will be unlikely to be able to repay the Covid-related loans they have taken during lockdown. A sad consequence will be many employers being unable to re-employ their previous numbers of staff and many businesses will cease trading. As is already happening, many more people will become unemployed.

The prospects for many young people entering the job market for the first time are bleak. Given that Covid-19 is predominantly a disease of older people, will all the young adhere to practices aimed at defending older people? Personally, I believe there is a good and healthy respect among the young for the wellbeing of older folk. However, it will become increasingly difficult to foster that good feeling when the life prospects of the young remain so bleak because of a disease predominantly affecting older people.

Commercial hardship in families will make it tougher for them to remain at home in social isolation. Poverty has always presented challenges for disease prevention schemes and the amount of new poverty we are likely to see in the UK this winter is quite alarming. Some of the people who are struggling to survive financially may be on hourly rate contracts with little or no pay during absenteeism. They often have little incentive to be officially tested for the coronavirus and feel more inclined to work on despite potential Covid symptoms.

Ironically those in work have considerable additional stresses which may be reflected in increased social activity and contact. This will be especially apparent in younger employees who will want to blow off steam in their social settings. That could include the drinking of alcohol and *any alcohol passing out of their blood into their lungs could increase the amount of virus breathed out by an infected person*.

When it comes to alcohol molecules weakening the protective mucus over the target cells and favouring replication of the coronavirus, it matters little whether the alcohol originates from beverages or hand sanitisers.

Autumn and winter are the seasons for common colds. People with overt Covid-19 symptoms are unlikely to be in any doubt they have a serious medical condition. However, many people are asymptomatic when they are infected by the coronavirus and these people will be spreading the virus. People with minor head colds or slight breathlessness but with no fever, cough or absence of taste or smell will have challenges in wondering whether they should consider the possibility that they are infected by the Covid coronavirus. If they decide to avoid being tested and actually are positive, they may transmit the virus through innocence.

In the UK we have been training people to avoid visiting their family doctor if they just have "a virus". A small fortune has been invested in telling people with sniffles to stay away from their GP as the latter lack any treatment for common colds. This winter a proportion of people suffering from a winter cold will actually be shedders of the coronavirus. They may adhere to the advice of having a coronavirus test done, although that will be hard to keep doing if a person has repeat episodes. I have considerable expertise in this field and I wonder how well I will be able to interpret a very low level of symptoms.

In the UK we choose to avoid enforced isolation of infected people or their contacts. We ask them to go into self-regulated isolation. Compare that with other countries where isolation is rigorously enforced, literally to the point of having people watching the corridors to prevent someone who might spread the virus leaving their home. Strict enforced isolation is very expensive to achieve and, in the current catastrophic economic situation, the UK may simply lack the resources to go that far. Or we may simply continue to lack the cultural will to do isolation as well as other nations. One thing is certain: we'll know soon enough what our lax isolation policy delivers.

That is a long list of reasons why I believe the UK is destined for a disastrous Covid-19 winter if we choose to continue as we are at the moment. The only factor I can influence is the use of alcohol sanitisers. That's why I've invested so much valuable time in writing this book.

There is some good news. It feels good to be writing that after the previous chapter.

CHAPTER 18

The Covid coronavirus is an RNA virus, and the RNA genetic code tends to allow for more little changes every time a virus particle is made. That is how the SARS virus progressively adapted into SARS-2 over all those years.

The good news is that experts can look at samples of virus from one setting and tell whether there have been multiple sources of the virus; whether that setting has been infected more than once. I recall one report where they could prove the virus had entered a care home on four separate occasions from four different sources. In due course that level of amazing finesse will help them identify weaknesses in our virus control procedures. It is by definition something that can only happen after the event, although even that is good news since it can help identify and eliminate sources of virus.

Combining that with an improving track and trace capacity will help curtail the virus.

If we are really lucky, a vaccine will save the day. Unfortunately, few people seem to believe a vaccine can be in widespread use in time for this winter. However, in dire times like these any glimmer of hope becomes valuable.

We are blessed with numerous potential vaccines entering clinical trials. Each vaccine needs to be proven effective and all the vaccine companies must find sufficient test subjects to prove efficacy claims. There are actually comparatively few test subjects for all their needs and the more vaccines there are in late stage development, the harder it will be to find enough test subjects. It is conceivable that we could have so many trial vaccines that they end up slowing each other down.

When a vaccine developed under the strict EU / UK protocols is available, I believe we will be safe and protected by that vaccine.

How long the immunity lasts is something only time can tell us.

Sadly we now return to the gloom of reality.

In my thesis the SARS virus settled into a form of balance by just infecting elderly people who had defective pulmonary surfactant protecting the lung cells that the virus attacked.

If my thesis is correct, the use of alcohol sanitisers generates solvent alcohol vapour which enters the lungs of elderly people with virus being replicated in their lungs. Those people would have subsequently produced many more virus particles than they would have done before the solvent vapour weakened even further their already weakened defences. In that scenario, the patients would have breathed out a lot more virus.

In time, the amount of airborne virus in the hospital setting will have become high enough to infect younger people, some of whom will have been healthcare workers.

That would signify a third level. First, the surfactant mucus defence was weakened by the elderly people being unable to make fully effective mucus. Second, the solvent vapours weakened the defences of those elderly patients further as a result of the simple chemical effect of dissolving parts of the mucus. The virus would have had easier access to the cells it attacked. Third, the number of virus particles required to infect a healthy healthcare worker would have become lower if that worker had solvent vapour in their alveolar air space. That in turn adds to the many more virus particles being breathed out by the patients in Covid wards.

Now the number of virus particles available to cause infection can best be assessed by the way this virus is spreading around the world. The necessity for frequent use of alcohol hand sanitisers may or may not be as relevant now to that rate of spread. At some point the number of virus particles could become high enough to produce new infections in their own right, without assistance from solvent vapours. Alcohol vapours would facilitate virus replication and spread, although, in some settings, the high virus count could reach the threshold where the virus can infect regardless of the vapour. Whether or not this proves to be the case remains to be confirmed.

Or we may be facing a combination in which the solvent vapour rising from alcohol sanitisers is helping the virus increase its numbers and the latter are leading to infection of the next person even without the new victim being affected by solvent vapours.

If the latter is correct, we need to pay particular attention to healthcare workers in Covid wards where we have people known to be infected and likely to be shedding the virus into their surroundings. That is the very space occupied by healthcare workers.

Anyone who continues to allow the use of alcohol hand sanitisers in Covid wards is gambling with the lives of both Covid-19 patients and the healthcare workers tending them, and therefore the population at large. This book puts the debate into the public domain. If the debate confirms my hypothesis, there will be interested parties who will seek redress against anyone who allowed this gamble to continue. Every death will become ammunition and there will be a time for the litigation spree.

Now is the time to come together against a common foe.

We have let the genie out of the bottle and it will not go back. Pursuing that analogy, there is simply too much virus to fit back in the original bottle. Nature had the virus in balance and we enabled it to multiply exponentially and out of any natural proportion. We provided the means for it to become pandemic.

Another useful analogy is to say we allowed the virus to spread like a wildfire. We then proceeded to use flammable alcohol as our favoured means of putting out the fire. Needless to say, the alcohol simply feeds the fire, and we earn ourselves an entirely unnatural global pandemic.

In global terms we still have a very naive population. Even though millions of people have become infected, that is a tiny proportion of the billions of people available to become infected. If we continue to fuel the fire with a flammable solvent we are indeed playing with fire for very high stakes. Hundreds of thousands have died. What will it take to prevent that from becoming millions of deaths? Hopefully, one small clue about alcohol sanitisers being recognised and acted upon.

In my view, national governments need now urgently to take the proactive step of reducing the solvent vapours that may have favoured excessive replication and spread of this coronavirus. That means substituting any products that result in solvent vapours entering the lungs. Alcohol sanitisers are the most commonly discussed source.

Others include strong disinfectants with volatile ingredients. In times as frightening as these, it is natural and common for scared people to reach for what they perceive to be the most powerful disinfectants. The assessment of strength can all too often be based on a stronger smell meaning the greater strength. Ironically that could be completely false. Some of the odourless products actually provide the best protection. However, if the smell is due to a solvent vapour, the high-odour disinfectant could be enabling the coronavirus to penetrate and infect the lung cells in the same way as alcohol vapour.

Many national governments are under a metaphorical siege by the virus. They are in a true state of paranoia about the coronavirus. Coronoia prevails.

It would be very unwise for the public to sit back and complain about their governments. You will have seen that although this book contains a lot of material arguing against the use of alcohol sanitisers, it also contains a lot of reasons why we will all benefit from the UK Cabinet appreciating it has one more choice. I have invested months in attempting to have that positive message reach the UK Cabinet. I have failed and there's a good chance I will continue to fail, unless the public weigh in to the campaign.

We might then win by sheer force of numbers. Or we might be fortunate that someone who can influence the Cabinet appreciates the simple message and its real import.

The government of any nation will suffice for our purposes of halting the pandemic spread. Most governments are members of the WHO and any government could effectively bring the simple message to the WHO.

I'm naming the UK Cabinet as my favoured route to political change because I live in the UK. If you are based elsewhere it will be interesting to hear how you progress. We have a global pandemic which makes it appropriate for the public around the world to do all they can.

CHAPTER 19

A lot of national leaders are distressed over the Covid-19 pandemic and the resultant economic calamity. They have a lot to do. Some are taking a posturing stance, saying the coronavirus is of little concern. Others will be reeling from the economic damage the pandemic is doing to their likelihood of success in future elections. Some will primarily be upset by the huge number of deaths. All of them will know the longer term legacy will be the absolutely huge cost in the medical care needed to help Covid survivors recover. In nations where the State covers that cost, the politicians will have a very serious economic challenge long after the pandemic has run its course.

One choice of action is to blame the politicians; another is to help them. It is unlikely that any of them could possibly have known this was going to happen when they chose to offer themselves for election to office. None of them can have been fully ready. Each of us shares the dilemma and all of us have a chance to help. I believe this book is one way I can help.

The worst option is for those in power to see me as someone they can completely ignore. Then I cannot help. So far the UK Cabinet members appear to have chosen this option. The failure even to acknowledge my emails is sending that message. The latter suggests that I am something and someone they can ignore. If there were no Covid-19 deaths, if I was without any success in defeating viruses, and if the economy was buoyant, it would not matter and it would be safe to leave the Cabinet to do whatever they are doing.

Sadly, since there are many thousands of Covid deaths, since I do bring a unique track record of having been able to render safe the threat posed by some viruses that the Cabinet's medical advisors are failing to overcome, and since the economy is in a mess and is heading for much worse, I would dearly like them to listen.

If you are a person who would like them to listen too, to you or me, then I am happy to be providing you with this book.

There are standard traditional ways to reach the UK Cabinet. If these were standard and traditional times we would all know what to do and how to do it. The fact that these times have no precedent creates an urgency that we use our freedom to find new ways of providing a positive contribution.

It is fun to see some of the many plausible conspiracy theories on social media. I may choose to use some of them in a novel should I opt to write a novel on this topic. However, at this point in time I would really prefer it if the resources in time and money being put into those conspiracy theories could be used to help the governments help the WHO help us all.

Every person reading this book will have something to offer. Some will see their role as being one in which they must apportion blame, either because that is the easier choice or because they feel the necessary action will only come from the relevant people and organisations feeling the pressure of blame. Even though I believe I'm offering a very positive and creative way forward, based on solid science, the title of this book shows that I believe that the WHO failed to tell us something and, so far, that the UK Cabinet has refused to hear. In one regard that could be seen as apportioning blame. However, I choose to see it as more than that; I see it as inducing movement. Should those two organisations prefer to remain intransigent I will leave others to reinforce blame. I will be using my resources somewhere else to present choices to real people facing real and present risk, with my desire being to induce therapeutic and potentially life-saving change.

If your government is choosing to ignore your contribution, how do you feel? Will you choose the view of your being such an insignificant member of the public that the people in authority really have more important things to worry about? If that is your view you are partly right; they do have other things to worry about. Yet I question any view of your being insignificant. In an earlier chapter, you read of the need for public momentum being the key to changing government actions. In generating the necessary momentum, the key lies in a lot of people each doing a very small amount. In reading this book you have taken valuable action. Others will gauge the level of momentum by things like how many people read this book and what they say in reviews. When sufficient people have taken that action, the book will be playing its part. So even though you may feel relatively insignificant in being just one of over 60 million UK residents, you are one that *can* make a difference.

The skill in generating public momentum lies in beginning with one. Then adding another one. You can see where that leads and you can be part of something very big and helpful.

Many people will be offering choices. We are all lucky in one way, in that we're living during an episode in which almost everyone wants to progress and see an end to the problem. In times like these it becomes much easier to amalgamate all the positive choices. This is part of my contribution. It is one of many. When enough individuals strive to progress towards one objective we build momentum.

Governments respect momentum. Some leaders will fight back against it and if you live under such a regime you can still gain from advances elsewhere.

CHAPTER 20

This book is the first time I have publicly used the word Coronoia. I want the word to symbolise a drive on from the depths of despair brought on by coronavirus paranoia and all its problems. I have taken steps to trademark Coronoia and in due course I anticipate an ® symbol will soon appear with the word.

Coronoia is the rallying word for constructive change around the world. Billions of people are currently affected by the pandemic in both health and economic ways.

The global Coronoia campaign is beginning in the UK because I live in England. Already people I know in other nations are adding their local contributions. It is a positive inclusive campaign in which we discover and bring forward constructive suggestions. Millions of people have good ideas and simply lack the means of having those ideas reach the people of influence and power.

We are offering a route for those wonderful ideas. Each progressive idea will attract more like-minded people to the campaign. Most politicians will begin to sense and value the positive momentum. We want them to open their minds to the many excellent ideas. We can expect there to be far too many good ideas for the few politicians to consider in depth, which is why we in the campaign will be compiling the ideas in ways that are simple to communicate.

Questions are often the best way to communicate. I've long held the view that the right answers are out there and all I need do is find the right questions. Another good way to communicate is to remain silent so others have their chance to present their ideas. Some of those ideas will be, or develop into, enlightened questions. When you lead with humility it is wonderful to see how many people want to join. Some of the questions for which I am best known have been shared with me by others. Since my aim is to find and to share the answers, I am always thrilled to make sure that people know where many of the brilliant questions I'm passing on actually arose.

Together we will present questions. Some will be intended to guide more like-minded people to join the campaign so they can better bring their ideas to the attention of others. These like-minded folk will benefit from safety in numbers. It is much easier to present and share a far-reaching idea when you are involved in a positive movement.

Some of the questions will be intended to induce comments from politicians. The word *Coronoia* adequately demonstrates what a sad state the world is in, and the word *campaign* shows we are seeking advancement from that mess. We happen to be in a positive progressive campaign so politicians will readily see we are offering them choices. They can continue to feel the fear which created the paranoia. That is their right and if they opt for that choice, it will have had, and will continue to have, implications on how they used the resources they had available at the time. There is also the chance that they could opt to use the Coronoia campaign to further their own agenda and so do everything they can to thwart our efforts. Any such action would allow us to demonstrate our momentum and show we are moving forward whether they want it or not. History shows how people who stand in front of a large moving mass often come to a metaphorical sticky end. That would be unfortunate as every politician has something to add. They are people after all, and we are building the Coronoia campaign on the belief that every person has something to offer. We want them to be relaxed in having their ideas shared by the campaign.

Some politicians will appreciate the benefit of being actively involved in a winning campaign. They are welcome as every politician comes with a large number of supporters. In parliamentary democracies, each politician also has many people who voted against them, and our task is to show those many people how much can be gained by their still joining the campaign.

Questions are the basis on which the Coronoia campaign is built. The campaign will end when the pandemic ends. As soon as the coronavirus paranoia subsides, our job will be complete. All those who have been willing to share their individual ideas, contributions and momentum can feel the rewarding feelings of having done something worthwhile for humanity and the planet.

There will be other matters to address, things like the environment and poverty. Both are being adversely affected by the pandemic. There was an initial environmental benefit in reduced emissions when travel was curtailed, yet we know now that may be short-lived. It's certain the environment is needing to deal with the massive amounts of single-use personal protective equipment. Food in shops is more likely to be wrapped in plastic to avoid people touching it. Poverty is increasing as economies suffer. So there will be plenty of good things to do when we disband this campaign. Effort put into ending Coronoia can then be used as good experience to address other global issues.

That is why joining the campaign now and seeing your good ideas translated into focused questions about Covid-19 actually generates and contributes to a long-term legacy.

You will be provided with questions to ask your political representative. You will know that the same question is being asked by many others in the campaign, avoiding any reason for you to stand out from the crowd. You will have safety in numbers.

You will also learn how few people need to ask the same question for UK politicians to take notice. Questions coming via the Coronoia campaign will be known as questions asked in order to achieve a positive progressive outcome. Accompanying our questions will be a discussion on how and why the politicians can benefit from the outcomes.

Politicians are smart and we have the advantage of knowing most of them favour being re-elected. The fact that the Coronoia campaign questions will be known to be constructive questions, means that any politician who chooses to not act for the benefit of their constituents will be seen to be taking an "interesting" political stance. They are allowed to. We are allowed to vote them out. We would like to have been able to disband the campaign long before the next UK general election. Fortunately, what our UK politicians do now to either support or hinder our campaign for the general good, will be known by their voters at the next election.

We will be polite; yet we will apply pressure if that helps end Coronoia.

CHAPTER 21

A book of this type is expected to end with a dystopian view, a stark statement on what is expected to happen if things don't change. Even for a person like me who uses a lot of words, finding something to effectively scare people who are already suffering from justifiable paranoia is a challenge.

So I'll opt to add numbers as those available are truly shocking. In the UK, we have lost well in excess of 40,000 people to Covid-19 so far. That's 40,000 deaths that would not have happened if the coronavirus had remained in balance. If the virus had been left to nudge a few elderly people who were due to die from bacterial pneumonia into a slightly premature final phase, that would have been sad enough. It's hard to find a word to distinguish that level of sadness with what we have seen around the world. But that is history and most of us know what has happened.

What is going to happen next? As the pandemic wave passes through one country after another, the death graphs in many countries have shown better news. At the time of writing this work in late August 2020, the official statistics for one week reveal very few deaths attributed to Covid-19. It is being argued that we have done a wonderful job of saving the NHS and smoothing out the curve. Apparently we should be feeling good about our level of success.

Yet we know 94% of the UK population still remain susceptible to this coronavirus. That's over 63 million people who are just as susceptible to the virus as we all were in January 2020. What's very different now is how much more coronavirus is circulating which was not here in January.

I am also a novelist. If I was writing a new novel and I wanted to create a hypothetical way of killing a massive number of people to make a really scary story, I cannot imagine a better situation than the one we find ourselves in now. Just think of the horror my made-up story could create. Over 60 million people to infect in just the UK, a virus that is spreading like wildfire and the Government telling everyone to use a flammable solvent to douse the fire. Everything would be in place for me to have people dying all over the place. In fact it would make a fantastic horror film.

As a novelist I choose to ask one question. Who would believe such a story? Nobody. It is just too incredible. Who would believe a government would suggest people in the path of a pandemic respiratory virus should ensure there was ample solvent vapour in their lungs to assist the virus in killing people? Simply infecting them is not enough to kill them. It takes something more to have infected people die. You need to be sure the flammable solvent vapours would be present in the infected lungs so the infection went to its natural conclusion of death, shedding even more virus into the air as it does so. Except that such a conclusion is not natural. It's entirely unnatural. It is man made. It's artificial.

That makes the story unbelievable and, as a novelist, I would not use it in a novel. It's too incredible for a fictional story. It's better presented in a non-fiction factual book with relevant medical references to prove it's real. That is why *Coronoia* is in the form it is.

Surely the WHO and all our governments would make certain no flammable solvent vapours would be allowed in the lungs of susceptible members of the public and people already infected by a virus that would take every advantage of the solvent vapours?

Or perhaps it's *What the WHO failed to tell us and the UK Cabinet refused to hear*. That sentence might make a good subtitle for a non-fiction book; a book based on reality.

The UK suffered over 40,000 deaths when the only thing going in the virus's favour was the presence of solvent vapours in the lungs which could dissolve the mucus protecting the very cells this virus wanted to reach and attack. Agreed that's just my thesis, and you know I'm open to suggestions on anything else that was favouring the virus to the extent we have seen.

If we lost that many when there was really only one thing helping the virus, what will happen if we keep that one thing in place and heap a lot more useful factors on top? Why not end the lockdown, why not mix children from different family groups at school? Let's consider doing lots of things just to help the virus multiply to even greater levels, infect more people and kill more of the ones it has infected.

We ARE doing that and more. For several months I have been seen as a negative person when I suggested this winter could bring at least double everything we have seen so far. I was very careful to only espouse that view in private commercial groupings. I have been very careful to keep such negativity from the press and so far I have been successful. I have tried very hard to have the dystopian view reach the UK Cabinet in a quiet manner and as you know I have failed so far.

Then out of nowhere I hear it reported that the UK Cabinet has a worst-case scenario for this winter, even worse than the one I was so careful to avoid sharing in public. Whether the report is true or not has little relevance in this state of Coronoia. The figure fits the reality so we have even more justification in taking all the actions we can think of to prevent what is coming.

To help, let's say we are heading for 100,000 Covid-19-related deaths in the UK over the coming winter. That number lies between what I feared could happen based on what I know and what the Government apparently is dreading might happen based on what they know. They know a lot more of what is going on behind the scenes than I do, so it's reasonable they would opt for a higher figure.

So it's 100,000 deaths before spring 2021. A decent dystopian view by anyone's standards.

Of course that is just the UK.

Now consider what *should happen* if the debate on my thesis goes my way. Alcohol sanitisers will become known as being very dangerous in Covid-19 settings. If we are very fortunate and that happens before winter, the much heralded calamity may not occur. At least not to that extent, as there remain many people with comorbidities that render them more susceptible, and the general UK diet does not optimise the state of the immune system.

The one simple action of substituting solvent-producing hand sanitisers in hospitals would allow the UK Cabinet to be seen in a positive light. That action would even induce me to bring out edition two of this book with the subtitle:

> *What the WHO failed to tell us and the UK Cabinet grasped immediately.*

That wonderful wording is something I need your help to achieve.

BIBLIOGRAPHY

1. Luisada AA, Goldmann MA, Weil R. "Alcohol vapor by inhalation in the treatment of acute pulmonary odema." *Circulation*. Volume V. March, 1952: 363.

2. Farmer H. *The Reaper's Rainbow*. Cambridge, Cambridgeshire: Cause Publications; 2009. ISBN 978-0-9562144-0-9

3. Elliott P, Storr J, Jeanes A. *Infection Prevention and Control: Perceptions and Perspectives*. Boca Raton, Florida: CRC Press; 2016. ISBN 978-184619-989-9

4. Ahmed-Lecheheb D, Cunat L, Hartemann P, Hautemaniere A. "Dermal and pulmonary absorption of ethanol from alcohol-based hand rub." *J Hosp Infect*. 2012: 81: 31-5.

5. Arndt T, Schrofel S, Gussregen B, Stemmerich K. "Inhalation but not transdermal resorption of hand sanitiser ethanol causes positive ethyl glucuronide findings in urine." *Forensic Sci Int*. 2014: 237: 126-30.

6. Joshi PC, Guidot DM. "The alcoholic lung: Epidemiology, pathophysiology, and potential therapies." *Am J Physiol*. 2007: 292: L813-L823.

7. Simet SM, Sisson JH. "Alcohol's effect on lung health and immunity." *Alcohol Res*. 2015: 37: 199-208.

8. Jobst KA, Shostak D, Whitehouse PJ. "Diseases of Meaning, Manifestations of Health, and Metaphor." *J Alt Comp Medicine*. 1999: 5: 495-502.

9. Royal College of Physicians. https://www.rcplondon.ac.uk/guidelines-policy/dermatitis-occupational-aspects-management-2009. Download titled *Dermatitis: Summary leaflet for healthcare professionals*.

10. Santos VS, Gurgel RQ, Cuevas LE, Martins-filho PR. "Prolonged fecal shedding of SARS-CoV-2 in paediatric patients: A quantitative evidence synthesis." *J Pediatr Gastroenterol Nutr*. 2020:10:1097.

ABOUT THE AUTHOR

Dr Harley Farmer is a director at NewGenne Ltd, a company that he co-founded in 2001. NewGenne specialises in preventing infectious diseases and supplies leading hygiene products around the world. However, the team's main contribution, as it has been since the company began in Dr Harley's kitchen twenty years ago, is inclusive thinking - appreciating what others are thinking and working to help them to achieve a better outcome.

Having grown up in the Australian outback, a harsh environment containing many potential dangers, Dr Harley learnt from an early age to care for others and that prevention is better, safer and easier than cure. Thousands of premature deaths arise from hospital infections every year and, believing that most of those deaths are avoidable, Dr Harley and NewGenne are actively working to prevent them. This now applies to the hundreds of thousands of Covid-19 deaths as well.

Confidence, like care and inclusivity, is another of Dr Harley's values. Having spent a lot of time examining the options and deciding which value is most beneficial, confidence is something that Dr Harley sees as vital to his work. He also loves science, philosophy and debate, yet the tool he relies on most of all is common sense.

Dr Harley has authored this book to share the latest information currently available together with pure science from credible sources. With thousands of lives at risk, this science should not be ignored.

When not working to prevent infectious diseases, Dr Harley can be found cooperating with the parents of children with atopic eczema to offer a solution to this insidious skin condition, or writing one of his gripping and shockingly plausible novels.

Visit www.dr-harley.com to learn more, or to contact Dr Harley Farmer directly.

www.ingramcontent.com/pod-product-compliance
Lightning Source LLC
LaVergne TN
LVHW050609100826
845148LV00015B/3190

* 9 7 8 0 9 5 6 9 7 0 7 9 4 *